DIABETIC COOKING

DELICIOUS, LIGHT & EASY

Publications International, Ltd.

Nutritional Analysis: Linda R. Yoakam, M.S., R.D.

Front Cover Photography: Laurie Proffitt Photography

Pictured on the front cover: Cashew Chicken (*page 80*).
Pictured on the back cover (*top to bottom*): Turkey Burger (*page 6*), Pasta e Fagioli (*page 40*) and Cherry Cobbler (*page 108*).
Pictured on the table of contents (*top to bottom*): Mediterranean Chicken Kabobs (*page 54*) and Pork with Sweet Hungarian Paprika (*page 60*).

ISBN: 0-7853-1688-4

Manufactured in U.S.A.

8   7   6   5   4   3   2   1

Microwave Cooking: Microwave ovens vary in wattage. The microwave cooking times given in this publication are approximate. Use the cooking times as guidelines and check for doneness before adding more time. Consult manufacturer's instructions for suitable microwave-safe cooking dishes.

CONTENTS

FACTS ABOUT DIABETES

Low calorie, low fat, low cholesterol and low sodium—buzzwords of the decade and for a good reason. People today are more aware than ever before of the roles that diet and exercise play in maintaining a healthful lifestyle. For people with diabetes and their families, the positive impact good nutrition and physical activity have on well-being is very familiar. Diabetes is a disease that affects the body's ability to use glucose as a source of fuel. When glucose is improperly utilized, it can build up in the bloodstream, creating higher than normal blood sugar levels. Left unchecked, elevated blood sugar levels may lead to the development of more serious long-term complications like blindness and heart and kidney disease.

Not all cases of diabetes are alike. In fact, the disease presents itself in two very distinct forms—type I and type II. Development of diabetes during childhood or adolescence is typical of type I diabetes. These individuals are unable to make insulin, a hormone produced by the pancreas that moves glucose from the bloodstream into the body's cells, where it is used as a source of fuel. Daily injections of insulin, coupled with a balanced meal plan, are the focus of treatment.

People who develop type II diabetes, the more common form of the disease, are typically over the age of 40 and obese. These individuals produce insulin but the amount is insufficient to meet their needs or, their excess weight renders the hormone incapable of adequately performing its functions. Treatment includes balanced eating, moderate weight loss, exercise and, in extreme cases, oral hypoglycemic agents or insulin injections.

MAXIMIZE HEALTH, MINIMIZE COMPLICATIONS

Diabetes increases your risk of developing high blood pressure and high blood cholesterol levels. Over time, elevated levels may progress to more serious complications, including heart and kidney disease, stroke and hypertension.

In fact, research shows that individuals with diabetes are nineteen times more likely to develop kidney disease and four times more likely to suffer from heart disease or a stroke than people who do not have diabetes. While heredity plays a major role in the development of these complications, regular check-ups with your physician and registered dietitian to fine-tune treatment strategies are good ways to help minimize complications. Strategies for treatment vary among individuals, yet overall goals remain the same: achieving and maintaining near-normal blood sugar levels by balancing food intake, insulin and activity, achieving optimal blood cholesterol levels and improving overall health through good nutrition.

BALANCE IS THE KEY

Achieving optimal nutrition often requires lifestyle changes to balance the intake of nutrients. The U.S. Department of Agriculture and the U.S. Department of Health and Human Services developed the Dietary Guidelines to simplify the basics of balanced eating and to help all individuals develop healthful eating plans. Several of the guidelines follow but were adjusted to include the revised 1994 American Diabetes Association's Nutrition Recommendations. Because recommendations are broad, work with your physician and registered dietitian to personalize the guidelines to meet your specific needs.

Eat a variety of foods. Energy, protein, vitamins, minerals and fiber are essential for optimal health, but no one food contains them all. Including a wide range of foods in your diet and using fats and oils sparingly throughout the day are easy ways to consume all the nutrients your body needs. Carbohydrate should comprise between 45 and 55 percent of total calories, and protein should contribute between 10 and 20 percent.

Maintain a healthy weight. Excess weight can worsen your diabetes and encourage the development of more severe complications. Research shows that shedding 10 to 20 pounds is enough to initiate positive results for obese individuals. Combining a healthful eating plan with physical activity outlined by your health care team is the best medicine for maintaining a healthy weight.

Choose a diet low in fat, saturated fat and cholesterol. Fat has more than double the calories of an equal amount of protein or carbohydrate. Thus, diets low in fat make it easier to maintain a desirable weight and decrease the likelihood of developing high blood cholesterol levels. Limit fat to no more than 30 percent of total calories, saturated fat to no more than 10 percent of total calories and daily cholesterol to no more than 300 mg. The 30 percent of calories from fat goal applies to a total diet over time, not to a single food, serving of a recipe or meal.

Choose a diet with plenty of vegetables, fruits and grain products. Vitamins, minerals, fiber and complex carbohydrates abound in these low-fat food choices. Filling up on fiber leaves less room for fat and may produce a slight decrease in blood cholesterol levels. Antioxidants such as beta carotene and the vitamins C and E may protect against heart disease, while magnesium, phosphorous and calcium are minerals that may keep blood pressure levels under control.

Use sugars in moderation. The ban on sugar has been lifted for people with diabetes but it is not altogether gone. The new guidelines for simple sugar intake are based on scientific research that indicates that carbohydrate in the form of simple sugars does not raise blood sugar levels more rapidly than any other type of carbohydrate food. What is more important is the total amount of carbohydrate consumed, not the source. However, keep in mind that since simple sugars are loaded with calories, contain no vitamins and minerals and are linked to the development of cavities, it is still a good idea to limit your intake of simple sugars to no more than 25 percent of total carbohydrate.

Use salt and sodium in moderation. Some people with diabetes may be more sensitive to sodium than others, making them more susceptible to high blood pressure. Minimize this risk by limiting sodium intake to no more than 2,400 mg a day (about 1 teaspoon of salt) and choosing single food items with less than 400 mg of sodium and entrées with less than 800 mg of sodium per serving.

FACTS ABOUT THE FOOD

The recipes in this publication were designed with people with diabetes in mind. But all are based on the principles of sound nutrition as outlined by the Dietary Guidelines, making them perfect for the entire family. Though the recipes in this publication are not intended as a medically therapeutic program, nor as a substitute for medically approved meal plans for individuals with diabetes, they are low in calories, fat, sodium and cholesterol and will fit easily into an individualized meal plan designed by your physician, registered dietitian and you.

FACTS ABOUT THE EXCHANGES

The nutrition information that appears with each recipe was calculated by an independent nutrition consulting firm and the Dietary Exchanges are based on the Exchange Lists for Meal Planning developed by the American Diabetes Association/The American Dietetic Association. Every effort has been made to check the accuracy of these numbers. However, because numerous variables account for a wide range of values in certain foods, all analyses that appear in this book should be considered approximate.

- The analysis of each recipe includes all the ingredients that are listed in that recipe, except ingredients labeled as "optional" or "for garnish." Foods shown in photographs on the same serving plate and offered as "serve with" suggestions at the end of a recipe are not included.

- If a range is offered for an ingredient, the first amount given was used to calculate the nutrition information.

- If an ingredient is presented with an option ("2 cups hot cooked rice or noodles" for example), the first item listed was used to calculate the nutrition information.

- Meat should be trimmed of all visible fat since this is reflected in the nutritional analysis.

- In recipes calling for cooked rice or noodles, the analysis was based on rice or noodles that were prepared without added salt and fat.

- Most processed foods contain significant amounts of sodium, which is reflected in the analysis. Rinsing processed foods under cold running water for one minute eliminates up to 60 percent of added sodium.

SANDWICHES & SNACKS

Add flair to midday munching with this delicious collection of sandwiches and snacks. Brown-baggers will welcome the outstanding selection of take-along treats.

Turkey Burgers

1 pound ground turkey breast
1 cup whole wheat bread crumbs
1 egg white
½ teaspoon dried sage leaves
½ teaspoon dried marjoram leaves
¼ teaspoon salt
¼ teaspoon ground black pepper
1 teaspoon vegetable oil
4 whole grain sandwich rolls, split in half
¼ cup Cowpoke Barbecue Sauce (page 80)*

*Or substitute prepared barbecue sauce.

1. Combine turkey, bread crumbs, egg white, sage, marjoram, salt and pepper in large bowl until well blended. Shape into 4 patties.

2. Heat oil in large nonstick skillet over medium-high heat until hot. Add patties. Cook 10 minutes or until patties are no longer pink in center, turning once.

3. Place one patty on bottom half of each roll. Spoon 1 tablespoon Cowpoke Barbecue Sauce over top of each burger. Place tops of rolls over burgers. Serve with lettuce and tomato; garnish with carrot slices, if desired.

Makes 4 burgers

NUTRIENTS PER SERVING:

Calories	319	Dietary Fiber	2 g
% calories from fat	17	Protein	26 g
Total Fat	6 g	Calcium	116 mg
Saturated Fat	1 g	Iron	3 mg
Cholesterol	41 mg	Vitamin A	20 RE
Sodium	669 mg	Vitamin C	4 mg
Carbohydrate	40 g		

Dietary Exchanges per Serving: 2 Starch/Bread, 3 Lean Meat

Turkey Burger

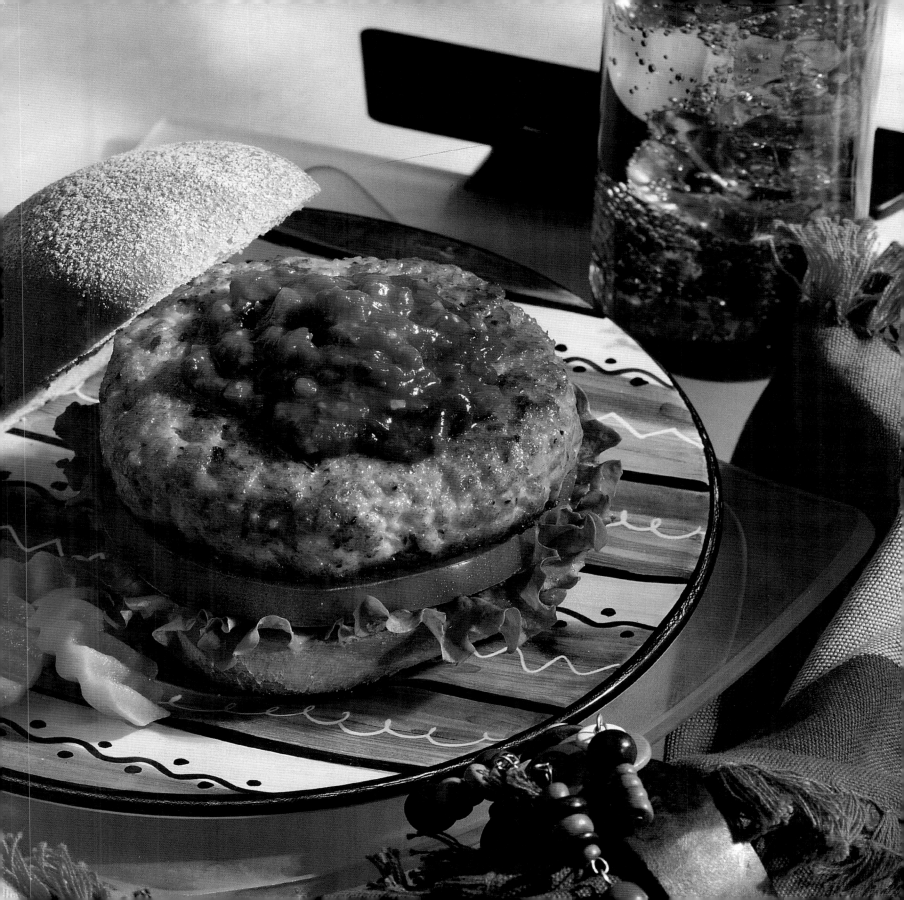

Mediterranean Vegetable Sandwiches

1 small eggplant, peeled, halved, cut into
¼-inch-thick slices
Salt
Nonstick cooking spray
1 small zucchini, halved, cut lengthwise into
¼-inch-thick slices
1 green or red bell pepper, sliced
3 tablespoons balsamic vinegar
½ teaspoon salt
½ teaspoon garlic powder
2 French bread rolls, halved

1. Place eggplant in non-aluminum colander; sprinkle eggplant with salt. Let stand 30 minutes to drain. Rinse eggplant; pat dry with paper towels.

2. Preheat broiler. Spray rack of broiler pan with nonstick cooking spray. Place vegetables on rack. Broil 4 inches from heat, 8 to 10 minutes or until vegetables are browned, turning once.

3. Blend vinegar, ½ teaspoon salt and garlic powder in medium bowl. Add vegetables; toss to coat. Divide vegetable mixture evenly between rolls. Garnish with apple slices, if desired. Serve immediately.

Makes 2 servings

NUTRIENTS PER SERVING:

Calories	178	Dietary Fiber	1 g
% calories from fat	10	Protein	5 g
Total Fat	2 g	Calcium	58 mg
Saturated Fat	<1 g	Iron	3 mg
Cholesterol	0 mg	Vitamin A	52 RE
Sodium	775 mg	Vitamin C	44 mg
Carbohydrate	36 g		

Dietary Exchanges per Serving: 1½ Starch/Bread, 3 Vegetable

Scrambled Egg Burritos

Nonstick cooking spray
1 red bell pepper, chopped
5 green onions, sliced
½ teaspoon crushed red pepper flakes
1 cup cholesterol-free egg substitute
1 tablespoon chopped fresh cilantro or parsley
4 (8-inch) flour tortillas
½ cup (2 ounces) shredded low-sodium
reduced-fat Monterey Jack cheese
⅓ cup salsa

1. Spray medium nonstick skillet with cooking spray. Heat over medium heat until hot. Add red pepper, onions and red pepper flakes. Cook and stir 3 minutes or until vegetables are crisp-tender.

2. Add egg substitute to vegetables. Reduce heat to low. Cook and stir 3 minutes or until set. Sprinkle with cilantro.

3. Stack tortillas and wrap in paper towels. Microwave at HIGH 1 minute or until tortillas are hot.

4. Place one fourth of egg mixture on each tortilla. Sprinkle with cheese. Fold sides over to enclose filling. Serve with salsa.

Makes 4 servings

NUTRIENTS PER SERVING:

Calories	186	Dietary Fiber	1 g
% calories from fat	20	Protein	14 g
Total Fat	4 g	Calcium	224 mg
Saturated Fat	1 g	Iron	3 mg
Cholesterol	6 mg	Vitamin A	422 RE
Sodium	425 mg	Vitamin C	27 mg
Carbohydrate	23 g		

Dietary Exchanges per Serving: 1 Starch/Bread, 1½ Lean Meat, 1 Vegetable

Mediterranean Vegetable Sandwich

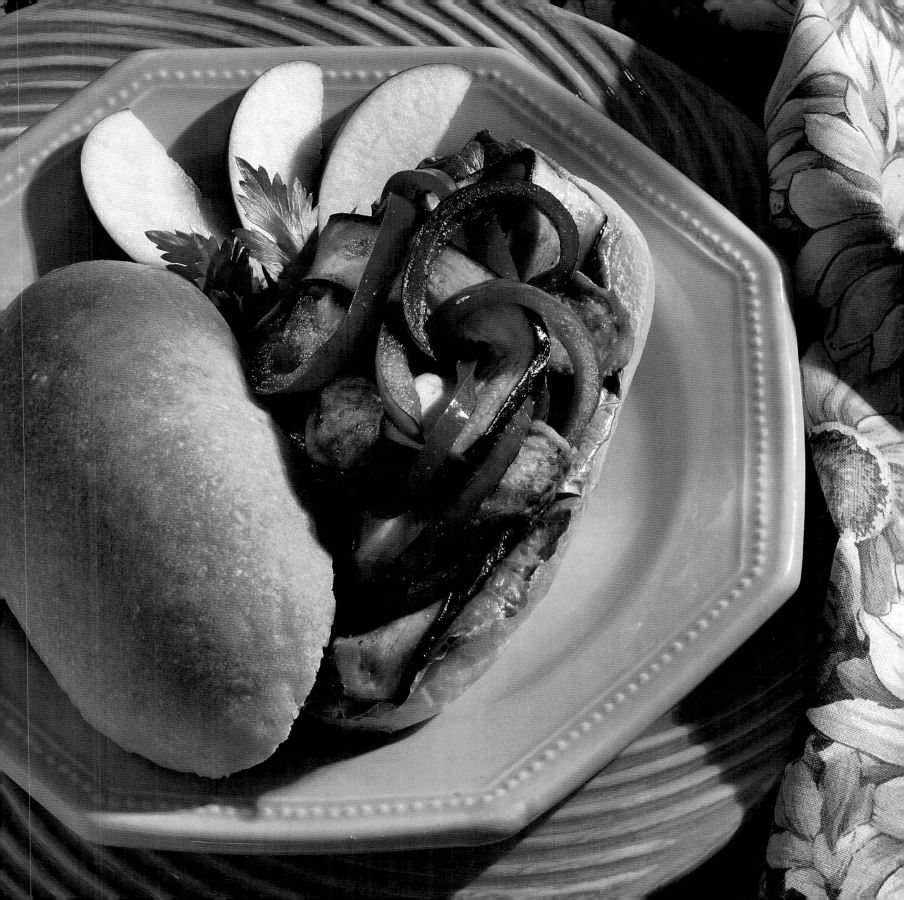

Bruschetta

Nonstick cooking spray
1 cup thinly sliced onion
½ cup chopped seeded tomato
2 tablespoons capers
¼ teaspoon black pepper
3 cloves garlic, finely chopped
1 teaspoon olive oil
4 slices French bread
½ cup (2 ounces) shredded reduced-fat
Monterey Jack cheese

1. Spray large skillet with cooking spray. Heat over medium heat until hot. Add onion. Cook and stir 5 minutes. Stir in tomato, capers and pepper. Cook 3 minutes.

2. Preheat broiler. Combine garlic and oil in small bowl; brush bread slices with mixture. Top with onion mixture; sprinkle with cheese. Place slices on baking sheet. Broil 3 minutes or until cheese melts.

Makes 4 servings

NUTRIENTS PER SERVING:

Calories	90	Dietary Fiber	<1 g
% calories from fat	20	Protein	3 g
Total Fat	2 g	Calcium	25 mg
Saturated Fat	<1 g	Iron	7 mg
Cholesterol	0 mg	Vitamin A	6 RE
Sodium	194 mg	Vitamin C	3 mg
Carbohydrate	17 g		

Dietary Exchanges per Serving: 1 Starch/Bread

California Rolls

1 cup reduced-fat ricotta cheese
2 (10-inch) flour tortillas
1 tomato, thinly sliced
2 cups torn spinach leaves
1 cup chopped onion
½ teaspoon dried oregano
½ teaspoon dried basil
1 cup alfalfa sprouts
4 ounces sliced turkey breast

Spread cheese evenly over tortillas to within ¼ inch of edges. Layer tomato, spinach, onion, oregano, basil, alfalfa sprouts and turkey over two-thirds of each tortilla. Roll up tortillas. Wrap in plastic wrap; refrigerate 1 hour. Cut crosswise into 10 slices.

Makes 4 servings

NUTRIENTS PER SERVING:

Calories	209	Dietary Fiber	2 g
% calories from fat	17	Protein	16 g
Total Fat	4 g	Calcium	132 mg
Saturated Fat	<1 g	Iron	3 mg
Cholesterol	28 mg	Vitamin A	233 RE
Sodium	233 mg	Vitamin C	17 mg
Carbohydrate	28 g		

Dietary Exchanges per Serving: 1½ Starch/Bread,
1½ Lean Meat, 1 Vegetable

Bruschetta

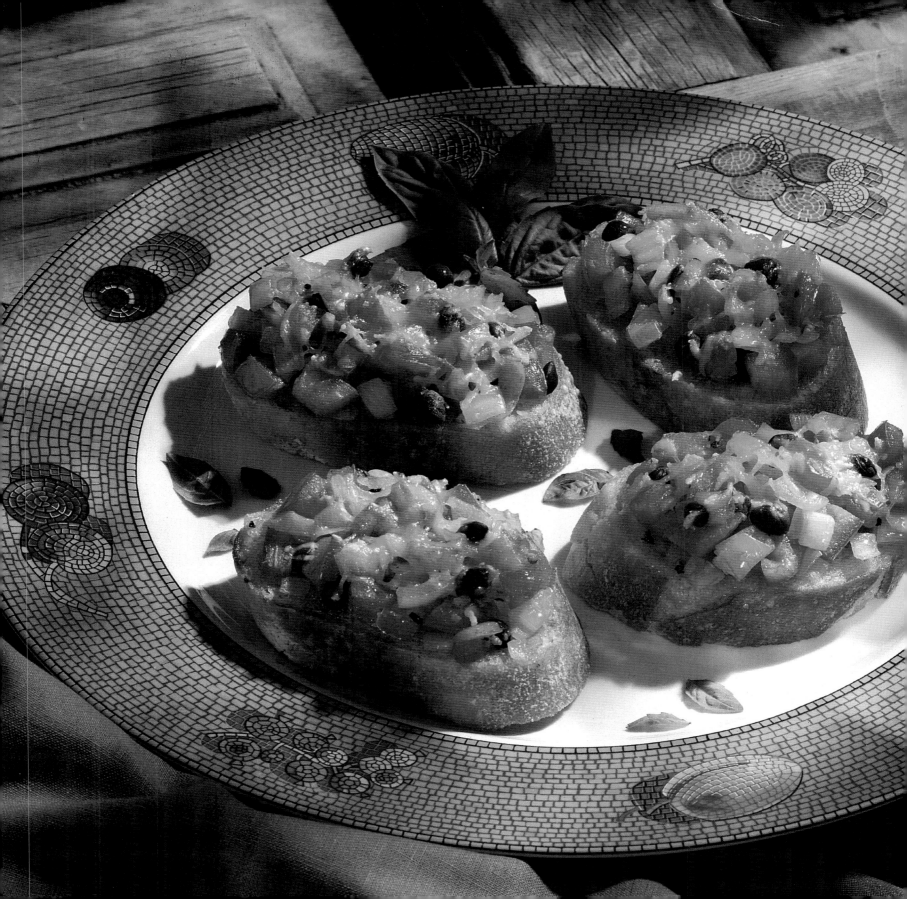

Roasted Eggplant Spread

1 large eggplant
1 can (14½ ounces) diced tomatoes, drained
½ cup finely chopped green onions
½ cup chopped fresh parsley
2 tablespoons red wine vinegar
1 tablespoon olive oil
3 cloves garlic, finely chopped
½ teaspoon salt
½ teaspoon dried oregano leaves
2 pita breads

1. Preheat oven to 375°F.

2. Place eggplant on baking sheet. Bake 1 hour or until tender, turning occasionally. Remove eggplant from oven. Let stand 10 minutes or until cool enough to handle.

3. Cut eggplant lengthwise in half; remove pulp. Place pulp in medium bowl; mash with fork until smooth. Add tomatoes, onions, parsley, vinegar, oil, garlic, salt and oregano; blend well. Cover eggplant mixture; refrigerate 2 hours.

4. Preheat broiler. Split pita breads horizontally in half to form 4 rounds. Stack rounds; cut into sixths to form 24 wedges. Place wedges on baking sheet. Broil 3 minutes or until crisp.

5. Serve eggplant mixture with warm pita bread wedges. Garnish with lemon and lime slices, if desired.

Makes 4 servings

NUTRIENTS PER SERVING:
6 pita bread wedges; ½ cup eggplant spread

Calories	134	Dietary Fiber	3 g
% calories from fat	20	Protein	4 g
Total Fat	3 g	Calcium	49 mg
Saturated Fat	<1 g	Iron	2 mg
Cholesterol	0 mg	Vitamin A	87 RE
Sodium	347 mg	Vitamin C	18 mg
Carbohydrate	23 g		

Dietary Exchanges per Serving: 1 Starch/Bread, 1 Vegetable, ½ Fat

South-of-the-Border Nachos

4 ounces low-fat tortilla chips
   Nonstick cooking spray
¾ cup chopped onion
2 jalapeño peppers, seeded, chopped*
3 cloves garlic, finely chopped
2 teaspoons chili powder
½ teaspoon ground cumin
1 boneless skinless chicken breast (about 6 ounces), cooked, chopped
1 can (14½ ounces) Mexican-style diced tomatoes, drained
1 cup (4 ounces) shredded reduced-fat Monterey Jack cheese
2 tablespoons black olives, chopped

*Jalapeño peppers can sting and irritate the skin. Wear rubber gloves when handling peppers and do not touch eyes.

1. Preheat oven to 350°F. Place chips in 13×9-inch baking pan.

2. Spray large nonstick skillet with cooking spray. Heat over medium heat until hot. Add onion, peppers, garlic, chili powder and cumin. Cook 5 minutes or until vegetables are tender, stirring occasionally. Stir in chicken and tomatoes.

3. Spoon tomato mixture, cheese and olives over chips. Bake 5 minutes or until cheese melts. Serve immediately.

Makes 4 servings

NUTRIENTS PER SERVING:

Calories	226	Dietary Fiber	2 g
% calories from fat	26	Protein	22 g
Total Fat	7 g	Calcium	377 mg
Saturated Fat	2 g	Iron	2 mg
Cholesterol	34 mg	Vitamin A	137 RE
Sodium	273 mg	Vitamin C	44 mg
Carbohydrate	21 g		

Dietary Exchanges per Serving: 1 Starch/Bread, 2 Lean Meat, 1 Vegetable, ½ Fat

Roasted Eggplant Spread

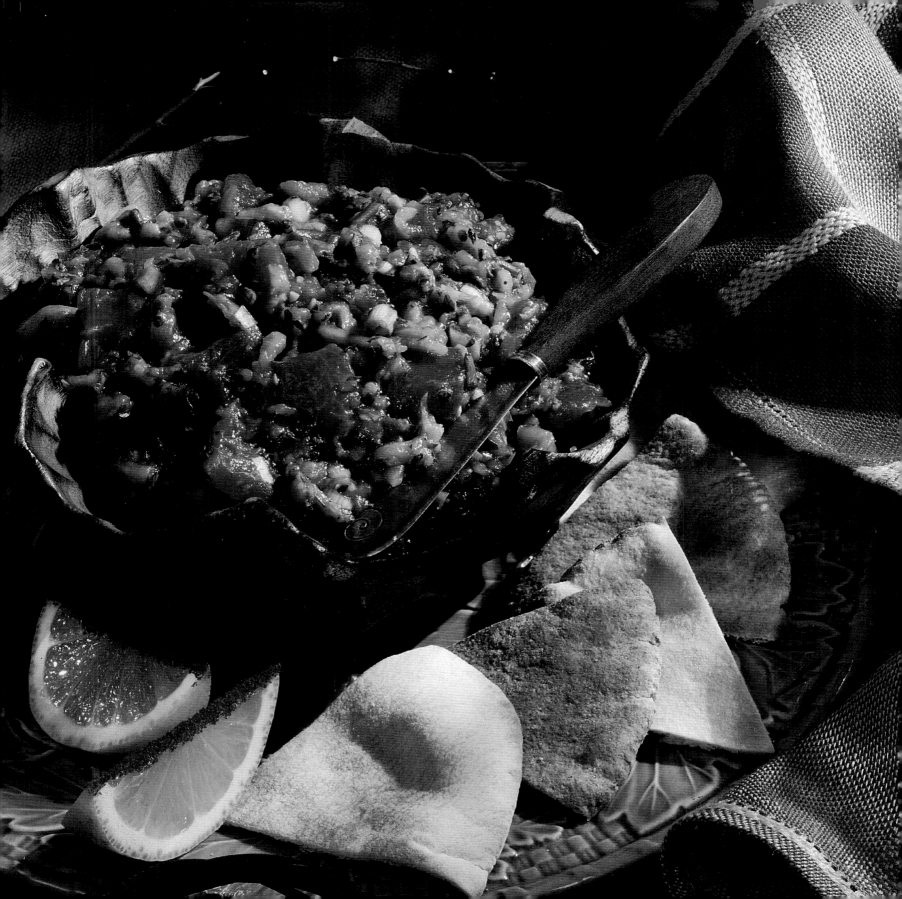

Tuna Salad Pita Pockets

1 (9-ounce) can tuna, drained
1 cup chopped cucumber
¼ cup part-skim ricotta cheese
2 tablespoons reduced-fat mayonnaise
2 tablespoons red wine vinegar
2 green onions, chopped
1 tablespoon sweet pickle relish
2 cloves garlic, finely chopped
½ teaspoon salt
¼ teaspoon black pepper
1 cup alfalfa sprouts
2 pita breads, halved

1. Combine tuna, cucumber, cheese, mayonnaise, vinegar, onions, relish, garlic, salt and pepper in medium bowl; blend well.

2. Divide sprouts evenly among pita bread halves. Spoon tuna mixture evenly into halves. Garnish with carrot strip and fresh herbs, if desired.

Makes 4 servings

NUTRIENTS PER SERVING:

Calories	209	Dietary Fiber	<1 g
% calories from fat	18	Protein	22 g
Total Fat	4 g	Calcium	55 mg
Saturated Fat	1 g	Iron	1 mg
Cholesterol	22 mg	Vitamin A	44 RE
Sodium	752 mg	Vitamin C	4 mg
Carbohydrate	22 g		

Dietary Exchanges per Serving: 1½ Starch/Bread, 2 Lean Meat

Cheesy Potato Skins

2 tablespoons grated Parmesan cheese
3 cloves garlic, finely chopped
2 teaspoons dried rosemary
½ teaspoon salt
¼ teaspoon black pepper
4 baked potatoes
2 egg whites, slightly beaten
½ cup (2 ounces) shredded part-skim mozzarella cheese

Preheat oven to 400°F. Combine Parmesan cheese and seasonings. Cut potatoes lengthwise in half. Remove pulp, leaving ¼-inch-thick shells. Cut shells lengthwise into wedges. Place wedges on baking sheet and brush with egg whites; sprinkle with cheese mixture. Bake 20 minutes. Sprinkle with mozzarella cheese; bake until melted. Serve with salsa, if desired.

Makes 8 servings

NUTRIENTS PER SERVING:

Calories	90	Dietary Fiber	2 g
% calories from fat	17	Protein	5 g
Total Fat	2 g	Calcium	85 mg
Saturated Fat	1 g	Iron	2 mg
Cholesterol	5 mg	Vitamin A	17 RE
Sodium	215 mg	Vitamin C	5 mg
Carbohydrate	14 g		

Dietary Exchanges per Serving: 1 Starch/Bread, ½ Lean Meat

Tuna Salad Pita Pocket

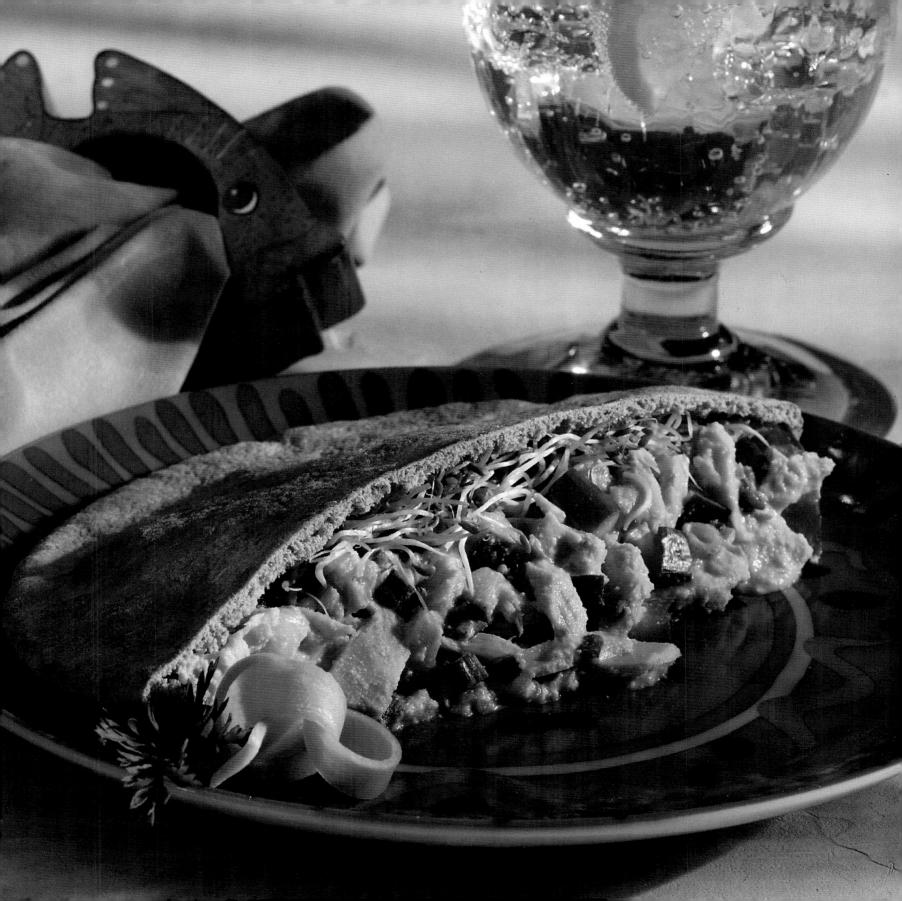

Black Bean Tostadas

1 cup rinsed, drained canned black beans, mashed
2 teaspoons chili powder
   Nonstick cooking spray
4 (6-inch) corn tortillas
1 cup washed, torn romaine lettuce leaves
1 cup chopped seeded tomato
½ cup chopped onion
½ cup plain nonfat yogurt
2 jalapeño peppers, seeded, finely chopped*

*Jalapeño peppers can sting and irritate the skin. Wear rubber gloves when handling peppers and do not touch eyes.

1. Combine beans and chili powder in small saucepan. Cook 5 minutes over medium heat or until heated through, stirring occasionally.

2. Spray large nonstick skillet with cooking spray. Heat over medium heat until hot. Sprinkle tortillas with water; place in skillet, one at a time. Cook 20 to 30 seconds or until hot and pliable, turning once.

3. Spread bean mixture evenly over tortillas; layer with lettuce, tomato, onion, yogurt and peppers. Garnish with cilantro, sliced tomatoes and peppers, if desired. Serve immediately. *Makes 4 servings*

NUTRIENTS PER SERVING:

Calories	146	Dietary Fiber	5 g
% calories from fat	9	Protein	9 g
Total Fat	2 g	Calcium	119 mg
Saturated Fat	<1 g	Iron	2 mg
Cholesterol	1 mg	Vitamin A	129 RE
Sodium	466 mg	Vitamin C	18 mg
Carbohydrate	29 g		

Dietary Exchanges per Serving: 1½ Starch/Bread, 1½ Vegetable

Hummus

1 can (about 15 ounces) garbanzo beans (chick-peas), rinsed and drained
3 tablespoons lemon juice
4½ teaspoons tahini*
½ teaspoon ground cumin
¼ teaspoon salt
¼ teaspoon ground black pepper
½ cup chopped seeded tomato
⅓ cup chopped red onion
⅓ cup chopped celery
⅓ cup chopped seeded cucumber
⅓ cup chopped green or red bell pepper
2 pita breads

*Tahini, a thick paste made from ground sesame seeds, is available in the ethnic section of major supermarkets, Middle Eastern markets or health food stores.

1. Combine beans, lemon juice, tahini, cumin, salt and black pepper in work bowl of food processor or blender container; process until smooth. If mixture is too thick to spread, add water until desired consistency is reached.

2. Spoon bean mixture into serving bowl. Top with tomato, onion, celery, cucumber and bell pepper.

3. Preheat broiler. Split pita breads horizontally in half to form 4 rounds. Stack rounds; cut into sixths to form 24 wedges. Place wedges on baking sheet. Broil 3 minutes or until crisp. Serve Hummus with warm pita bread wedges. *Makes 4 servings*

NUTRIENTS PER SERVING:
6 pita bread wedges, ½ cup Hummus

Calories	188	Dietary Fiber	4 g
% calories from fat	17	Protein	7 g
Total Fat	4 g	Calcium	69 mg
Saturated Fat	1 g	Iron	3 mg
Cholesterol	0 mg	Vitamin A	24 RE
Sodium	542 mg	Vitamin C	23 mg
Carbohydrate	33 g		

Dietary Exchanges per Serving: 2 Starch/Bread, ½ Vegetable, ½ Fat

Black Bean Tostada

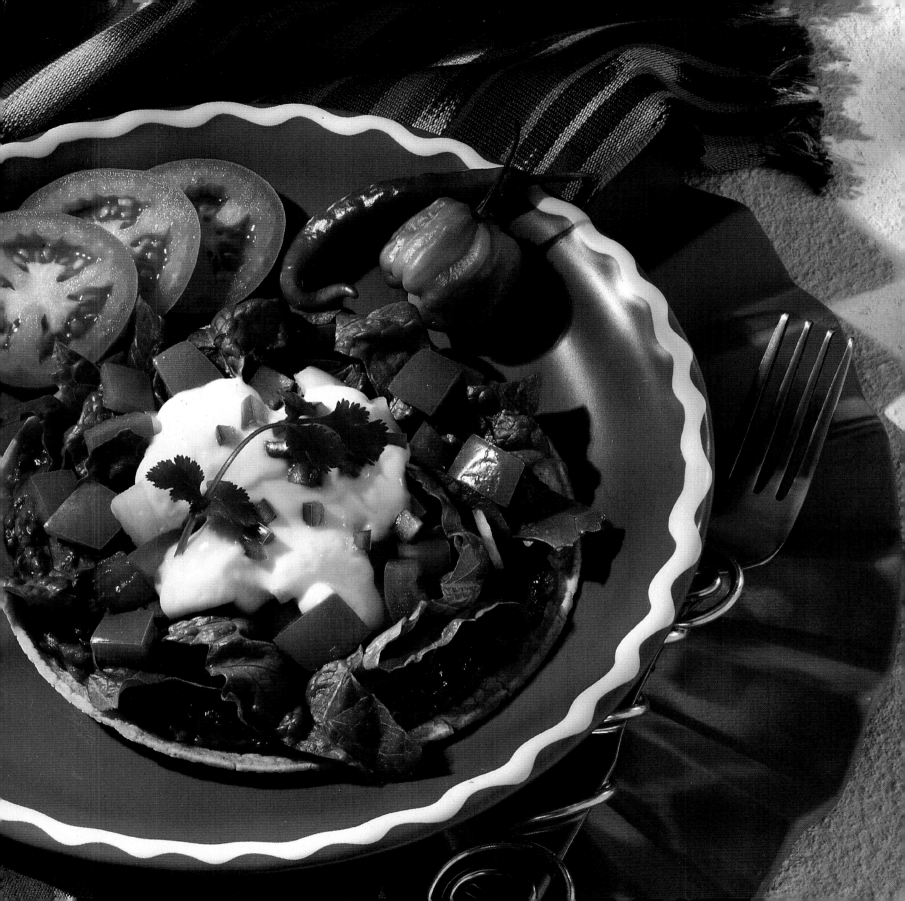

Miniature Fruit Muffins

1 cup whole wheat flour
¾ cup all-purpose flour
½ cup packed dark brown sugar
2 teaspoons baking powder
½ teaspoon baking soda
¼ teaspoon salt
1 cup buttermilk, divided
¾ cup frozen blueberries
1 small ripe banana, mashed
¼ teaspoon vanilla
⅓ cup unsweetened applesauce
2 tablespoons raisins
½ teaspoon ground cinnamon

1. Preheat oven to 400°F. Spray 36 miniature muffin cups with nonstick cooking spray; set aside.

2. Combine flours, sugar, baking powder, baking soda and salt in medium bowl. Place ⅓ of dry ingredients in each of 3 small bowls.

3. To one portion flour mixture, add ⅓ cup buttermilk and blueberries. Stir just until blended; spoon into 12 prepared muffin cups. To second portion, add ⅓ cup buttermilk, banana and vanilla. Stir just until blended; spoon into 12 more prepared muffin cups. To final portion, add remaining ⅓ cup buttermilk, applesauce, raisins and cinnamon. Stir just until blended; spoon into remaining 12 prepared muffin cups.

4. Bake 18 minutes or until lightly browned and wooden pick inserted into centers comes out clean. Remove from pan. Cool 10 minutes on wire racks. Serve warm or cool completely.   *Makes 12 servings*

NUTRIENTS PER SERVING: *3 miniature muffins*

Calories	130	Dietary Fiber	2 g
% calories from fat	4	Protein	3 g
Total Fat	1 g	Calcium	49 mg
Saturated Fat	<1 g	Iron	1 mg
Cholesterol	1 mg	Vitamin A	4 RE
Sodium	178 mg	Vitamin C	2 mg
Carbohydrate	29 g		

Dietary Exchanges per Serving: 1 Starch/Bread,
1 Fruit

Italian Stuffed Mushrooms

8 large mushrooms
  Nonstick cooking spray
2 ounces lean ground pork
½ cup whole wheat bread crumbs
1 egg white
2 green onions, finely chopped
1 teaspoon dried oregano leaves
¼ teaspoon ground black pepper
½ cup (2 ounces) shredded nonfat mozzarella
  cheese

1. Preheat oven to 350°F.

2. Remove stems from mushrooms; set caps aside. Finely chop stems.

3. Spray small nonstick skillet with cooking spray. Heat over medium heat until hot. Add chopped stems and pork. Cook and stir 5 minutes or until pork is no longer pink.

4. Combine pork mixture, bread crumbs, egg white, onions, oregano and pepper in medium bowl until well blended. Spoon pork mixture evenly into mushroom caps, mounding slightly in center. Place caps on baking sheet. Sprinkle cheese evenly over tops of mushrooms.

5. Bake 15 minutes or until mushrooms are tender. Serve immediately.   *Makes 4 servings*

NUTRIENTS PER SERVING:

Calories	69	Dietary Fiber	1 g
% calories from fat	16	Protein	10 g
Total Fat	1 g	Calcium	146 mg
Saturated Fat	<1 g	Iron	1 mg
Cholesterol	11 mg	Vitamin A	46 RE
Sodium	153 mg	Vitamin C	2 mg
Carbohydrate	5 g		

Dietary Exchanges per Serving: 1 Lean Meat,
1 Vegetable

Miniature Fruit Muffins

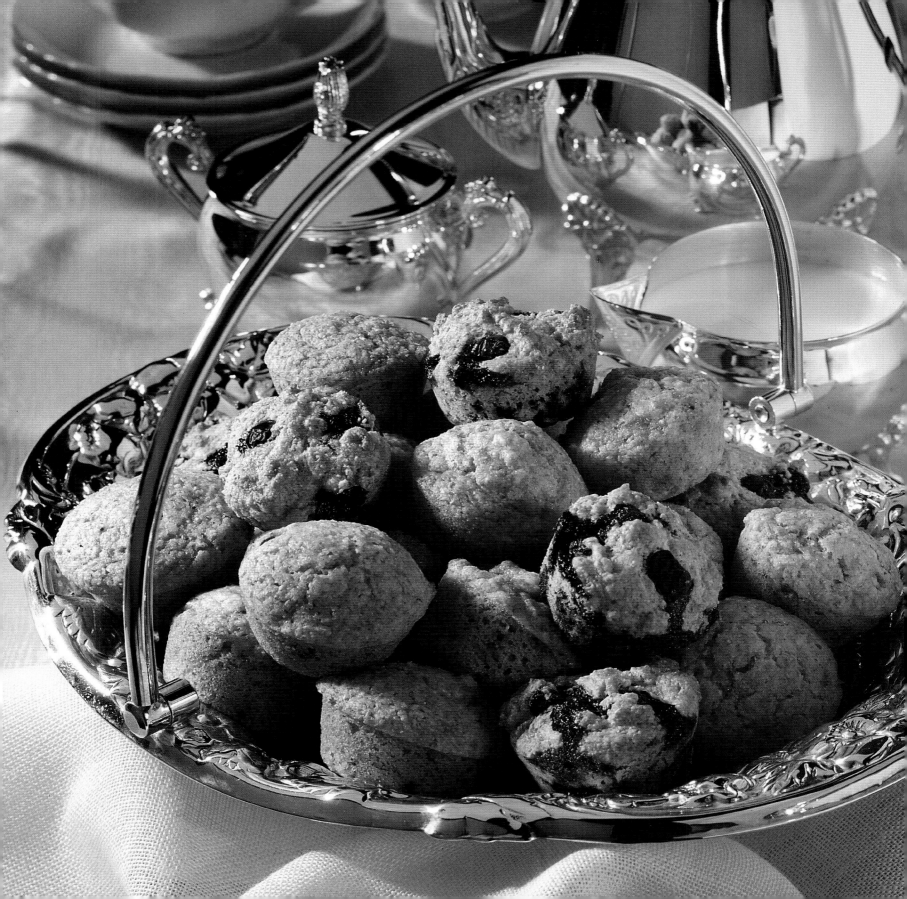

Bean & Cheese Quesadillas

Spicy Salsa (recipe follows)
½ cup nonfat ricotta cheese
4 (6-inch) flour tortillas
½ cup rinsed, drained pinto beans, cooked, mashed
½ cup (2 ounces) shredded reduced-fat Monterey Jack cheese

1. Prepare Spicy Salsa. Spread ricotta cheese evenly over half of each tortilla. Layer tortillas with beans, Monterey Jack cheese, and 2 tablespoons salsa. Fold in half.

2. Spray small nonstick skillet with nonstick cooking spray. Heat over medium-high heat until hot. Place tortillas in skillet, one at a time. Cook 4 minutes or until golden brown and cheese melts, turning once. Cut tortillas in half. Serve with remaining 1½ cups Spicy Salsa. *Makes 4 servings*

Spicy Salsa

1 cup chopped seeded tomato
¼ cup finely chopped green onions
¼ cup finely chopped fresh cilantro
2 tablespoons lime juice
1 jalapeño pepper, seeded, finely chopped*
2 cloves garlic, finely chopped

*Jalapeño peppers can sting and irritate the skin. Wear rubber gloves when handling peppers and do not touch eyes.

Combine all ingredients in small bowl until well blended. Let stand 1 hour. *Makes about 2 cups*

NUTRIENTS PER SERVING:

Calories	237	Dietary Fiber	3 g
% calories from fat	26	Protein	14 g
Total Fat	7 g	Calcium	235 mg
Saturated Fat	3 g	Iron	1 mg
Cholesterol	20 mg	Vitamin A	147 RE
Sodium	265 mg	Vitamin C	17 mg
Carbohydrate	31 g		

Dietary Exchanges per Serving: 2½ Starch/Bread, 1 Fat

Pepper-Cheese Polenta

¾ teaspoon sugar
¼ teaspoon salt
⅓ cup yellow or white cornmeal
¼ cup chopped red or green bell pepper
½ cup (2 ounces) shredded reduced-fat Monterey Jack cheese

1. Spray 8½×4½-inch loaf pan with nonstick cooking spray; set aside.

2. Combine 1 cup water, sugar and salt in small saucepan. Bring to a boil over high heat. Stir in cornmeal with wire whisk. Reduce heat to medium. Cook 10 minutes or until mixture thickens and pulls away from side of pan, stirring constantly.

3. Spoon polenta into prepared pan; cover. Refrigerate 1 hour or until firm.

4. Preheat broiler. Cut polenta into 4 slices. Sprinkle pepper and cheese evenly over slices. Place slices on baking sheet. Broil 3 to 5 minutes or until cheese melts. Serve immediately. *Makes 4 servings*

NUTRIENTS PER SERVING:

Calories	84	Dietary Fiber	2 g
% calories from fat	30	Protein	6 g
Total Fat	3 g	Calcium	129 mg
Saturated Fat	2 g	Iron	<1 mg
Cholesterol	10 mg	Vitamin A	44 RE
Sodium	249 mg	Vitamin C	13 mg
Carbohydrate	10 g		

Dietary Exchanges per Serving: ½ Starch/Bread, ½ Lean Meat, ½ Fat

Seafood Tacos with Fruit Salsa

Fruit Salsa (recipe follows)
2 tablespoons lemon juice
1 teaspoon chili powder
1 teaspoon ground allspice
1 teaspoon minced garlic
1 to 2 teaspoons grated lemon peel
1 teaspoon olive oil
½ teaspoon ground cloves
1 pound halibut or snapper fillets
12 (6-inch) corn tortillas *or* **6 (7- to 8-inch) flour tortillas**
3 cups washed and torn romaine lettuce leaves
1 small red onion, halved, thinly sliced

1. To prevent sticking, spray grill with nonstick cooking spray. Prepare coals for grilling.

2. Prepare Fruit Salsa; set aside.

3. Combine lemon juice, chili powder, allspice, garlic, lemon peel, oil and cloves in small bowl. Rub fish with spice mixture. (Fish may be cut into smaller pieces for easier handling.)

4. Place fish on grill. Grill, covered, 5 minutes or until fish is opaque in center and flakes easily when tested with fork, turning occasionally. Remove from heat; cut into 12 pieces, removing bones if necessary. Cover to keep warm.

5. Place tortillas on grill in single layer; cook 20 seconds or until hot and pliable, turning occasionally. Stack; cover to keep warm.

6. Top each tortilla with ¼ cup lettuce and red onion. Add 1 piece of fish and about 2 tablespoons Fruit Salsa. *Makes 6 servings*

NUTRIENTS PER SERVING: *1 taco, 2 tablespoons Fruit Salsa*

Calories	294	Dietary Fiber	6 g
% calories from fat	14	Protein	21 g
Total Fat	5 g	Calcium	162 mg
Saturated Fat	1 g	Iron	3 mg
Cholesterol	24 mg	Vitamin A	171 RE
Sodium	296 mg	Vitamin C	68 mg
Carbohydrate	43 g		

Dietary Exchanges per Serving: 1½ Starch/Bread, 2 Lean Meat, 1 Fruit, ½ Vegetable

Fruit Salsa

1 small ripe papaya, peeled, seeded, chopped
1 firm small banana, chopped
2 green onions, finely chopped
3 tablespoons chopped fresh cilantro or mint
3 tablespoons lime juice
2 jalapeño peppers, seeded, finely chopped*

*Jalapeño peppers can sting and irritate the skin; wear rubber gloves when handling peppers and do not touch eyes.

Combine all ingredients in small bowl. Serve at room temperature. *Makes 12 servings*

Health Note: Halibut is low in fat and also lower in cholesterol and sodium than many other kinds of fish.

Thai Chicken Pizzas

2 boneless skinless chicken breast halves
  (½ pound)
2 teaspoons Thai seasoning
  Nonstick cooking spray
2 tablespoons pineapple juice
1 tablespoon peanut butter
1 tablespoon oyster sauce
1 teaspoon Thai chili paste*
2 (10-inch) flour tortillas
½ cup shredded carrot
½ cup sliced green onions
½ cup red bell pepper slices
¼ cup chopped fresh cilantro
½ cup (2 ounces) shredded part-skim mozzarella
  cheese

*Thai chili paste is available at some larger supermarkets and at Oriental markets.

1. Preheat oven to 400°F. Cut chicken breasts crosswise into thin slices, each about 1½×½ inch. Sprinkle with Thai seasoning. Let stand 5 minutes. Spray large nonstick skillet with cooking spray; heat over medium heat until hot. Add chicken. Cook and stir 3 minutes or until chicken is no longer pink in center.

2. Blend pineapple juice, peanut butter, oyster sauce and chili paste in small bowl until smooth. Place tortillas on baking sheets. Spread peanut butter mixture over tortillas. Divide chicken, carrot, green onions, pepper and cilantro evenly between tortillas. Sprinkle with cheese. Bake 5 minutes or until tortillas are crisp and cheese is melted. Cut into wedges.

Makes 4 servings

NUTRIENTS PER SERVING:

Calories	201	Dietary Fiber	1 g
% calories from fat	31	Protein	18 g
Total Fat	7 g	Calcium	140 mg
Saturated Fat	2 g	Iron	2 mg
Cholesterol	38 mg	Vitamin A	655 RE
Sodium	556 mg	Vitamin C	71 mg
Carbohydrate	17 g		

Dietary Exchanges per Serving: 1 Starch/Bread, 2 Lean Meat, ½ Vegetable

Health Note: Beta-carotene, which is found in certain red, orange, yellow and green pigmented fruits and vegetables, is converted by the body into vitamin A. Carrots and red pepper combine in this recipe to provide more than half the Recommended Dietary Allowance of vitamin A.

Thai Chicken Pizzas

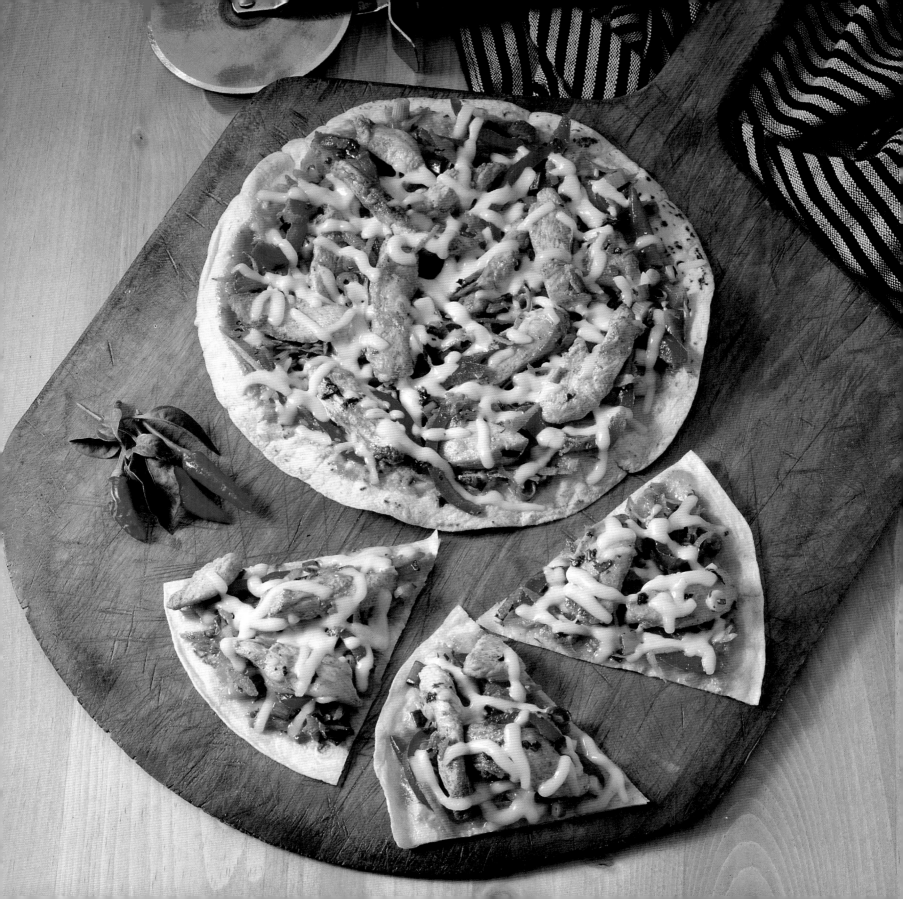

Meatless Sloppy Joes

Nonstick cooking spray
2 cups thinly sliced onions
2 cups chopped green peppers
2 cloves garlic, finely chopped
2 tablespoons ketchup
1 tablespoon mustard
1 can (about 15 ounces) kidney beans, mashed
1 can (8 ounces) tomato sauce
1 teaspoon chili powder
Cider vinegar
2 sandwich rolls, halved

1. Spray large nonstick skillet with cooking spray; heat over medium heat until hot. Add onions, peppers and garlic. Cook and stir 5 minutes or until vegetables are tender. Stir in ketchup and mustard.

2. Add beans, sauce and chili powder. Reduce heat to medium-low. Cook 5 minutes or until thickened, stirring frequently and adding up to ⅓ cup vinegar if dry. Top sandwich roll halves evenly with bean mixture.   *Makes 4 servings*

NUTRIENTS PER SERVING:

Calories	242	Dietary Fiber	10 g
% calories from fat	7	Protein	10 g
Total Fat	2 g	Calcium	102 mg
Saturated Fat	<1 g	Iron	3 mg
Cholesterol	0 mg	Vitamin A	158 RE
Sodium	994 mg	Vitamin C	113 mg
Carbohydrate	48 g		

Dietary Exchanges per Serving: 2 Starch/Bread,
3 Vegetable, ½ Fat

Trail Mix Truffles

⅓ cup dried apples
¼ cup dried apricots
¼ cup apple butter
2 tablespoons golden raisins
1 tablespoon reduced-fat peanut butter
½ cup low-fat granola
¼ cup graham cracker crumbs, divided
¼ cup mini chocolate chips

Blend fruit, apple butter, raisins and peanut butter in food processor until smooth. Stir in granola, 1 tablespoon crumbs, chips and 1 tablespoon water. Place remaining crumbs in bowl. Shape tablespoonfuls mixture into balls; roll in crumbs to coat. Cover; refrigerate until ready to serve.   *Makes 8 servings*

NUTRIENTS PER SERVING:

Calories	121	Dietary Fiber	2 g
% calories from fat	30	Protein	3 g
Total Fat	4 g	Calcium	49 mg
Saturated Fat	1 g	Iron	1 mg
Cholesterol	0 mg	Vitamin A	30 RE
Sodium	14 mg	Vitamin C	1 mg
Carbohydrate	20 g		

Dietary Exchanges per Serving: 1 Starch/Bread,
½ Fruit, ½ Fat

Meatless Sloppy Joe

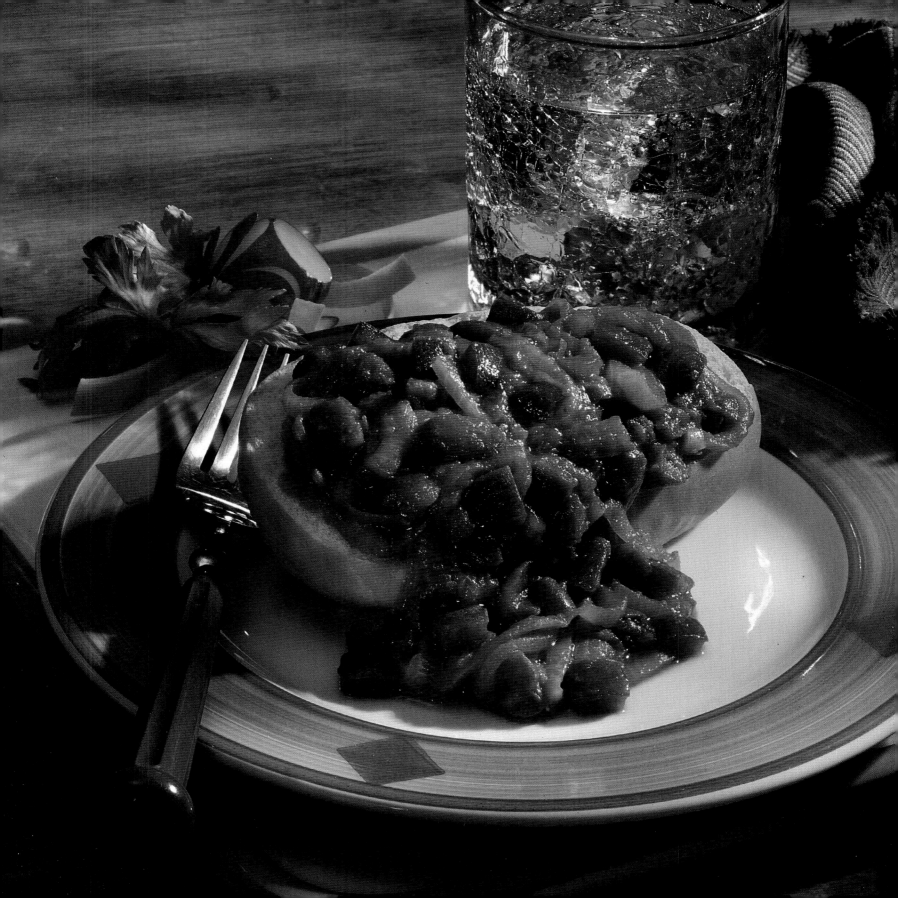

Turkey Gyros

     1 turkey tenderloin (8 ounces)
 1½ teaspoons Greek seasoning
     1 cucumber
  ⅔ cup plain nonfat yogurt
  ¼ cup finely chopped onion
     2 teaspoons dried dill weed
     2 teaspoons fresh lemon juice
     1 teaspoon olive oil
     4 pita breads
 1½ cups washed and shredded romaine lettuce
     1 tomato, thinly sliced
     2 tablespoons crumbled feta cheese

1. Cut turkey tenderloin across the grain into ¼-inch slices. Place turkey slices on plate; lightly sprinkle both sides with Greek seasoning. Let stand 5 minutes.

2. Cut two thirds of cucumber into thin slices. Finely chop remaining cucumber. Combine chopped cucumber, yogurt, onion, dill weed and lemon juice in small bowl.

3. Heat olive oil in large skillet over medium heat until hot. Add turkey. Cook 2 minutes on each side or until cooked through. Wrap 2 pita breads in paper toweling. Microwave at HIGH 30 seconds or just until warmed. Repeat with remaining pita breads. Divide lettuce, tomato, cucumber slices, turkey, cheese and yogurt-cucumber sauce evenly among pita breads; fold edges over and secure with wooden picks.

Makes 4 servings

NUTRIENTS PER SERVING:

Calories	319	Dietary Fiber	1 g
% calories from fat	12	Protein	27 g
Total Fat	4 g	Calcium	205 mg
Saturated Fat	2 g	Iron	3 mg
Cholesterol	55 mg	Vitamin A	101 RE
Sodium	477 mg	Vitamin C	17 mg
Carbohydrate	42 g		

Dietary Exchanges per Serving: 2½ Starch/Bread, 2 Lean Meat, 1 Vegetable

Tarragon Chicken Salad Sandwiches

 1¼ pounds boneless skinless chicken breasts, cooked
     1 cup thinly sliced celery
     1 cup seedless red or green grapes, cut into halves
  ½ cup raisins
  ½ cup plain nonfat yogurt
  ¼ cup reduced-fat mayonnaise or salad dressing
     2 tablespoons finely chopped shallots or onion
     2 tablespoons minced fresh tarragon *or*
        1 teaspoon dried tarragon leaves
  ½ teaspoon salt
  ⅛ teaspoon white pepper
     6 lettuce leaves
     6 whole wheat buns, split

1. Cut chicken into scant ½-inch pieces. Combine chicken, celery, grapes and raisins in large bowl. Blend yogurt, mayonnaise, shallots, tarragon, salt and pepper in small bowl. Spoon over chicken mixture; mix lightly.

2. Place 1 lettuce leaf in each bun. Divide chicken mixture evenly; spoon into buns.   *Makes 6 servings*

NUTRIENTS PER SERVING:

Calories	353	Dietary Fiber	4 g
% calories from fat	18	Protein	34 g
Total Fat	7 g	Calcium	120 mg
Saturated Fat	1 g	Iron	2 mg
Cholesterol	76 mg	Vitamin A	62 RE
Sodium	509 mg	Vitamin C	6 mg
Carbohydrate	41 g		

Dietary Exchanges per Serving: 1½ Starch/Bread, 4 Lean Meat, ½ Fruit

Turkey Gyro

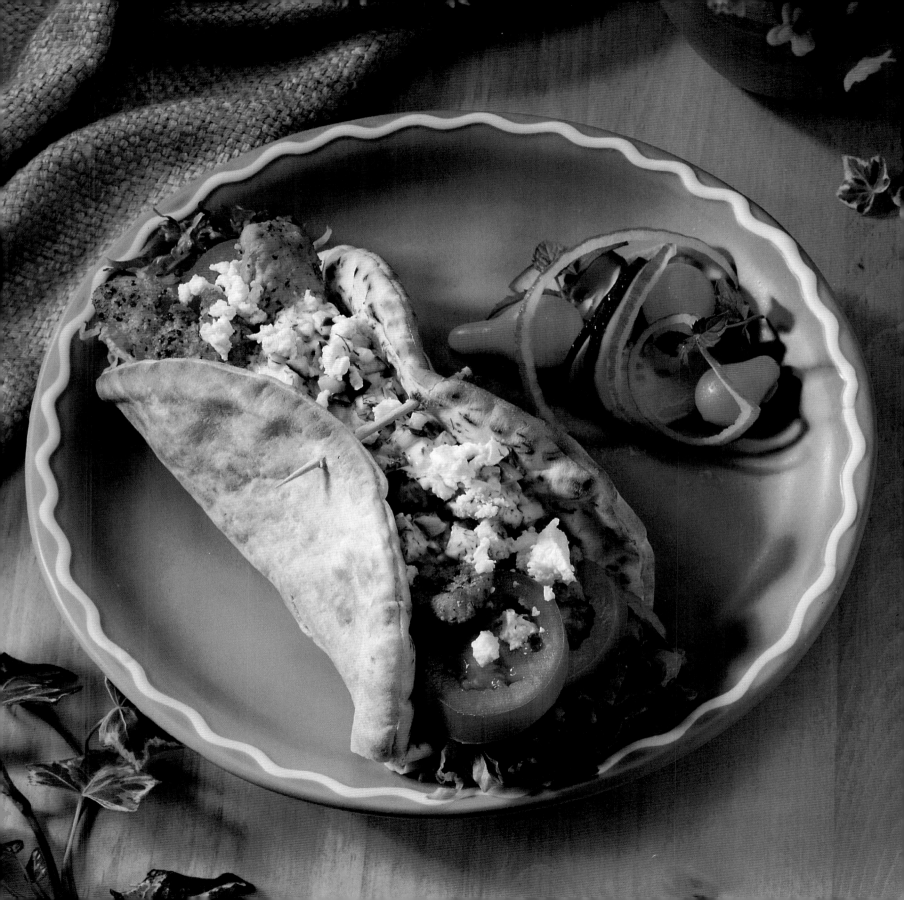

SUPER SOUPS & SALADS

Crunch your way through crispy salads or spoon into splendid soups for a refreshing change of pace. Enjoy them on their own or as an appetizing prelude to a meal.

Apple Slaw with Poppy Seed Dressing

1 cup coarsely chopped unpeeled Jonathan apple
1 teaspoon lemon juice
2 tablespoons nonfat sour cream
4½ teaspoons skim milk
1 tablespoon frozen apple juice concentrate, thawed
1 teaspoon sugar
¾ teaspoon poppy seeds
½ cup sliced carrots
⅓ cup shredded green cabbage
⅓ cup shredded red cabbage
2 tablespoons finely chopped green bell pepper
Additional cabbage leaves (optional)

1. Combine apple and lemon juice in small bowl; toss to coat.

2. Blend sour cream, milk, apple juice concentrate, sugar and poppy seeds in small bowl. Add apple mixture, carrots, cabbages and pepper; toss to coat. Serve on additional cabbage leaves and garnish with fresh greens and carrot slice, if desired.   *Makes 2 servings*

NUTRIENTS PER SERVING:

Calories	94	Dietary Fiber	2 g
% calories from fat	7	Protein	3 g
Total Fat	1 g	Calcium	92 mg
Saturated Fat	<1 g	Iron	1 mg
Cholesterol	<1 mg	Vitamin A	375 RE
Sodium	34 mg	Vitamin C	44 mg
Carbohydrate	21 g		

Dietary Exchanges per Serving: 1 Fruit, 1 Vegetable

Apple Slaw with Poppy Seed Dressing

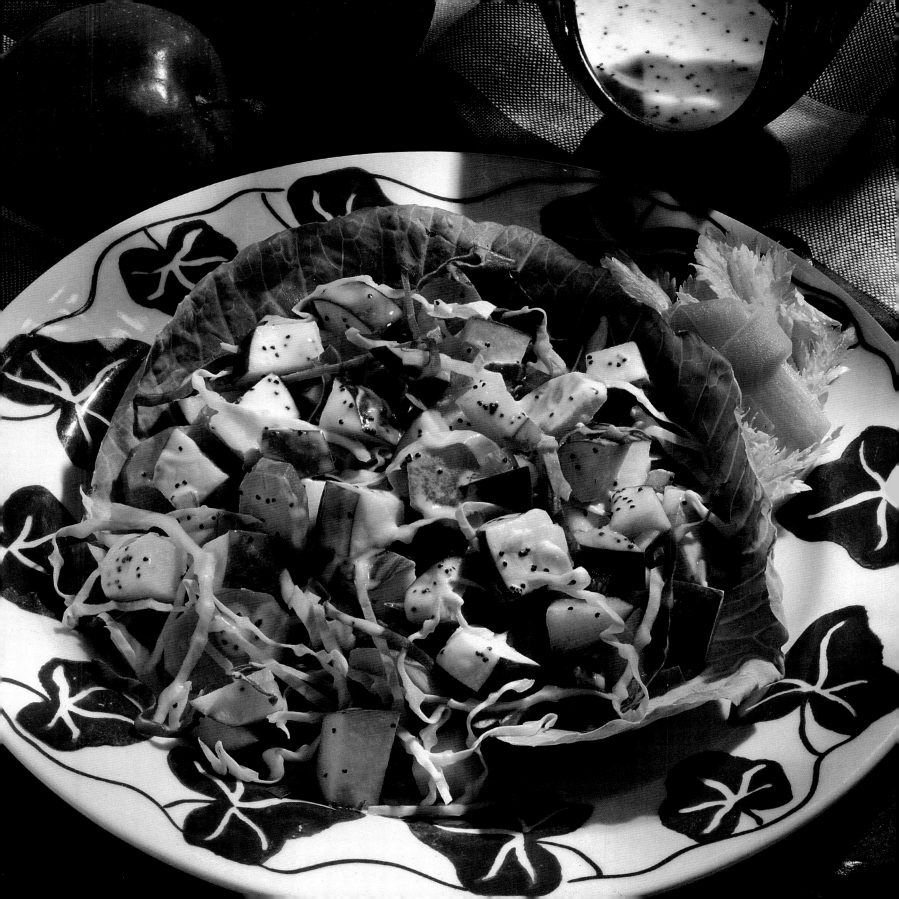

Vegetarian Chili

1 tablespoon vegetable oil
2 cloves garlic, finely chopped
1½ cups thinly sliced mushrooms
⅔ cup chopped red onion
⅔ cup chopped red bell pepper
2 teaspoons chili powder
¼ teaspoon ground cumin
⅛ teaspoon ground red pepper
⅛ teaspoon dried oregano leaves
1 can (28 ounces) peeled whole tomatoes
⅔ cup frozen baby lima beans
½ cup rinsed, drained canned Great Northern beans
3 tablespoons nonfat sour cream
3 tablespoons shredded reduced-fat Cheddar cheese

1. Heat oil in large nonstick saucepan over medium-high heat until hot. Add garlic. Cook and stir 3 minutes. Add mushrooms, onion and bell pepper. Cook 5 minutes, stirring occasionally. Add chili powder, cumin, ground red pepper and oregano. Cook and stir 1 minute. Add tomatoes and beans. Reduce heat to medium-low. Simmer 15 minutes, stirring occasionally.

2. Top servings evenly with sour cream and cheese.

Makes 4 servings

NUTRIENTS PER SERVING:

Calories	189	Dietary Fiber	7 g
% calories from fat	24	Protein	10 g
Total Fat	5 g	Calcium	154 mg
Saturated Fat	1 g	Iron	4 mg
Cholesterol	3 mg	Vitamin A	467 RE
Sodium	428 mg	Vitamin C	121 mg
Carbohydrate	29 g		

Dietary Exchanges per Serving: 1 Starch/Bread, 3 Vegetable, 1 Fat

Hot Chinese Chicken Salad

¼ cup fat-free reduced-sodium chicken broth
2 tablespoons reduced-sodium soy sauce
2 tablespoons rice wine vinegar
1 tablespoon rice wine or dry sherry
1 teaspoon sugar
½ teaspoon crushed red pepper
1 tablespoon vegetable oil, divided
1½ cups fresh pea pods, sliced diagonally
1 cup thinly sliced green or red bell pepper
1 clove garlic, finely chopped
1 pound boneless skinless chicken breasts, cut into ½-inch pieces
1 cup thinly sliced red or green cabbage
8 ounces fresh or steamed Chinese egg noodles, cooked
2 green onions, thinly sliced

1. Blend chicken broth, soy sauce, vinegar, rice wine, sugar and crushed red pepper in small bowl; set aside.

2. Heat 1 teaspoon oil in large nonstick skillet or wok. Add pea pods, bell pepper and garlic. Cook 1 to 2 minutes or until vegetables are crisp-tender; set aside. Heat remaining 2 teaspoons oil in skillet. Add chicken; cook 3 to 4 minutes or until chicken is no longer pink. Add cabbage, cooked vegetables and noodles. Stir in sauce; toss to coat evenly. Cook and stir 1 to 2 minutes or until heated through. Sprinkle with green onions before serving. *Makes 6 servings*

NUTRIENTS PER SERVING:

Calories	164	Dietary Fiber	2 g
% calories from fat	30	Protein	17 g
Total Fat	6 g	Calcium	34 mg
Saturated Fat	1 g	Iron	2 mg
Cholesterol	45 mg	Vitamin A	81 RE
Sodium	353 mg	Vitamin C	55 mg
Carbohydrate	12 g		

Dietary Exchanges per Serving: ½ Starch/Bread, 2 Lean Meat, 1 Vegetable, ½ Fat

Vegetarian Chili

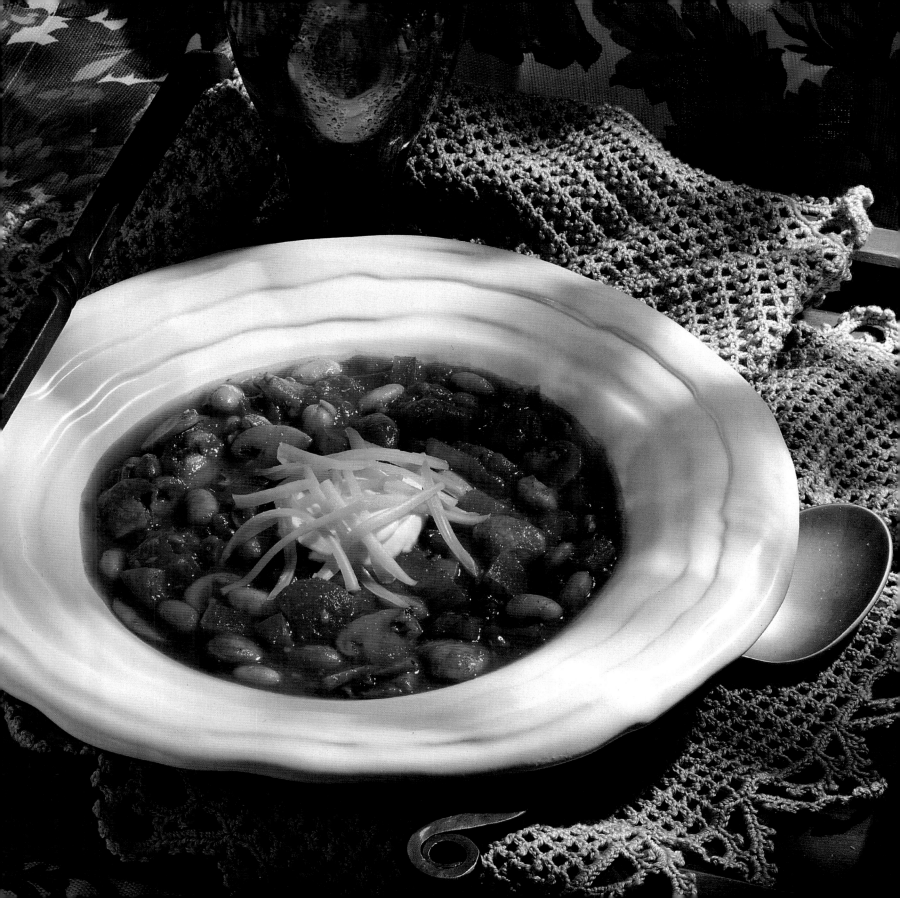

Zesty Taco Salad

    2 tablespoons vegetable oil
    1 clove garlic, finely chopped
    ¾ pound ground turkey
    1¾ teaspoons chili powder
    ¼ teaspoon ground cumin
    3 cups washed, torn lettuce leaves
    1 can (14½ ounces) Mexican-style diced
        tomatoes, drained
    1 cup rinsed, drained canned garbanzo beans
        (chick-peas) or pinto beans
    ⅔ cup chopped peeled cucumber
    ⅓ cup frozen whole kernel corn, thawed
    ¼ cup chopped red onion
    1 to 2 jalapeño peppers, seeded, finely
        chopped* (optional)
    1 tablespoon red wine vinegar
    12 nonfat tortilla chips
        Fresh greens (optional)

* Jalapeño peppers can sting and irritate the skin. Wear rubber gloves when handling peppers and do not touch eyes.

1. Combine oil and garlic in small bowl; let stand 1 hour. Combine turkey, chili powder and cumin in large nonstick skillet. Cook over medium heat 5 minutes or until no longer pink, stirring to crumble.

2. Combine turkey, lettuce, tomatoes, beans, cucumber, corn, onion and jalapeño in large bowl. Remove garlic from oil; discard garlic. Blend oil and vinegar. Drizzle over salad; toss to coat. Serve on tortilla chips and fresh greens, if desired. Serve with additional tortilla chips and garnish with cilantro, if desired.   *Makes 4 servings*

NUTRIENTS PER SERVING:

Calories	285	Dietary Fiber	5 g
% calories from fat	33	Protein	21 g
Total Fat	11 g	Calcium	77 mg
Saturated Fat	1 g	Iron	3 mg
Cholesterol	33 mg	Vitamin A	123 RE
Sodium	484 mg	Vitamin C	23 mg
Carbohydrate	28 g		

Dietary Exchanges per Serving: 1½ Starch/Bread, 2 Lean Meat, 1 Vegetable, 1 Fat

Waldorf Salad

    1 unpeeled tart red apple, such as McIntosh,
        coarsely chopped
    1 teaspoon fresh lemon juice
    4 teaspoons frozen apple juice concentrate,
        thawed
    1 tablespoon fat-free mayonnaise
    1 tablespoon nonfat sour cream
    ⅛ teaspoon paprika
    ½ cup finely chopped celery
    6 large lettuce leaves, washed
    5 teaspoons coarsely chopped walnuts

1. Combine apple and lemon juice in resealable plastic food storage bag. Seal bag; toss to coat.

2. Combine apple juice concentrate, mayonnaise, sour cream and paprika in medium bowl until well blended. Add apple mixture and celery; toss to coat. Cover; refrigerate 2 hours before serving.

3. Serve each salad over lettuce leaves. Top each serving evenly with walnuts.   *Makes 2 servings*

NUTRIENTS PER SERVING:

Calories	115	Dietary Fiber	3 g
% calories from fat	30	Protein	3 g
Total Fat	4 g	Calcium	43 mg
Saturated Fat	<1 g	Iron	1 mg
Cholesterol	0 mg	Vitamin A	65 RE
Sodium	134 mg	Vitamin C	25 mg
Carbohydrate	19 g		

Dietary Exchanges per Serving: 1 Fruit, 1 Fat

Zesty Taco Salad

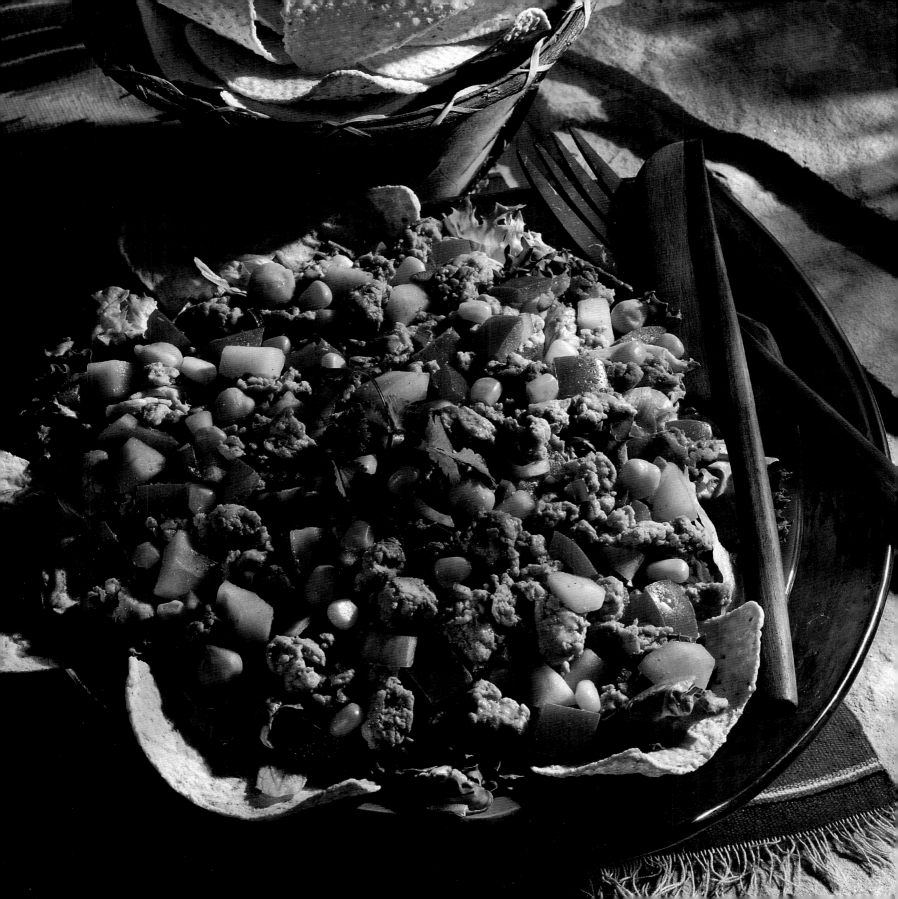

Clam Chowder

1 can (5 ounces) whole baby clams, undrained
1 potato, peeled, coarsely chopped
¼ cup finely chopped onion
⅔ cup evaporated skim milk
    Pinch ground white pepper
    Pinch dried thyme leaves
1 tablespoon reduced-calorie margarine

1. Drain clams; reserve juice. Add enough water to reserved juice to measure ⅔ cup. Combine clam juice mixture, potato and onion in large saucepan. Bring to a boil over high heat. Reduce heat to medium-low. Simmer 8 minutes or until potato is tender.

2. Add milk, pepper and thyme to saucepan. Increase heat to medium-high. Cook and stir 2 minutes. Add margarine. Cook 5 minutes or until soup thickens, stirring occasionally. Stir in clams. Cook 5 minutes or until clams are firm, stirring occasionally. Garnish with red pepper strip, thyme and greens, if desired.

Makes 2 servings

NUTRIENTS PER SERVING:

Calories	204	Dietary Fiber	1 g
% calories from fat	17	Protein	14 g
Total Fat	4 g	Calcium	295 mg
Saturated Fat	1 g	Iron	3 mg
Cholesterol	47 mg	Vitamin A	164 RE
Sodium	205 mg	Vitamin C	9 mg
Carbohydrate	30 g		

Dietary Exchanges per Serving: 1 Starch/Bread, 1 Lean Meat, 1 Milk

Health Note: A meal plan high in dietary calcium may actually prevent—not promote—the formation of kidney stones. Studies indicate that calcium, abundant in foods like milk, yogurt, cottage cheese and ricotta cheese, appears to bind oxalates that are linked to the formation of the stones.

Thai Pasta Salad with Peanut Sauce

¼ cup evaporated skim milk
4½ teaspoons creamy peanut butter
4½ teaspoons finely chopped red onion
1 teaspoon lemon juice
¾ teaspoon brown sugar
½ teaspoon reduced-sodium soy sauce
⅛ teaspoon crushed red pepper
½ teaspoon finely chopped fresh ginger
1 cup hot cooked whole wheat spaghetti
2 teaspoons finely chopped green onion

1. Combine milk, peanut butter, red onion, lemon juice, sugar, soy sauce and red pepper in medium saucepan. Bring to a boil over high heat, stirring constantly. Boil 2 minutes, stirring constantly. Reduce heat to medium-low. Add ginger; blend well. Add spaghetti; toss to coat.

2. Top servings evenly with green onion. Serve immediately.

Makes 2 servings

NUTRIENTS PER SERVING:

Calories	187	Dietary Fiber	3 g
% calories from fat	26	Protein	9 g
Total Fat	6 g	Calcium	111 mg
Saturated Fat	1 g	Iron	1 mg
Cholesterol	38 mg	Vitamin A	45 RE
Sodium	85 mg	Vitamin C	3 mg
Carbohydrate	27 g		

Dietary Exchanges per Serving: 1½ Starch/Bread, ½ Milk, 1 Fat

Clam Chowder

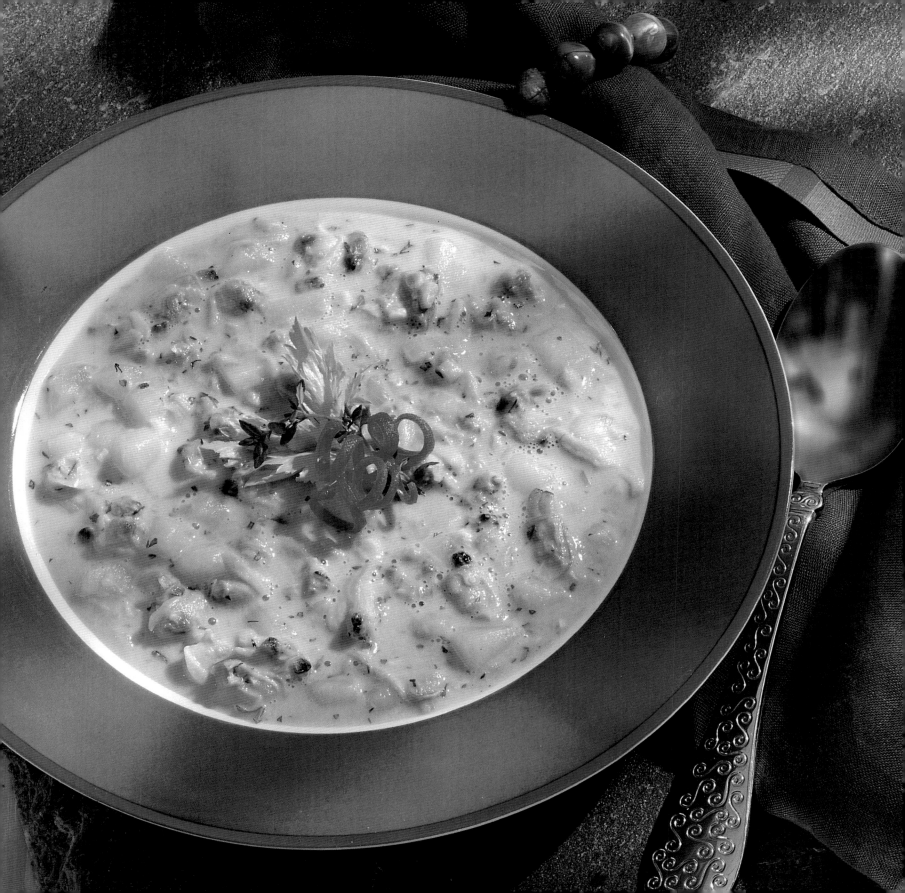

Taos Chicken Salad

Lime Vinaigrette (recipe follows)
3 flour or corn tortillas, cut into ¼-inch strips
Nonstick cooking spray
1 pound boneless skinless chicken thighs, cut into strips
6 cups washed and torn assorted salad greens
2 oranges, peeled and cut into segments
2 cups peeled jicama strips
1 can (about 15½ ounces) pinto beans, rinsed and drained
1 cup cubed red bell pepper
½ cup sliced celery
½ cup sliced green onions with tops

1. Prepare Lime Vinaigrette; set aside. Preheat oven to 350°F. Spray tortilla strips lightly with cooking spray; place in 15×10-inch jelly-roll pan. Bake about 10 minutes or until browned, stirring occasionally. Cool to room temperature.

2. Spray medium nonstick skillet with cooking spray; heat over medium heat until hot. Add chicken; cook and stir about 15 minutes or until no longer pink in center. Refrigerate until chilled.

3. Combine greens, oranges, jicama, beans, pepper, celery and green onions in large bowl; add chicken. Drizzle with Lime Vinaigrette; toss to coat. Serve immediately; garnish with tortilla strips.

Makes 6 servings

NUTRIENTS PER SERVING:

Calories	258	Dietary Fiber	6 g
% calories from fat	19	Protein	18 g
Total Fat	6 g	Calcium	143 mg
Saturated Fat	1 g	Iron	4 mg
Cholesterol	37 mg	Vitamin A	281 RE
Sodium	437 mg	Vitamin C	100 mg
Carbohydrate	36 g		

Dietary Exchanges per Serving: 1½ Starch/Bread, 1½ Lean Meat, ½ Fruit, 1 Vegetable

Lime Vinaigrette

3 tablespoons finely chopped fresh cilantro or parsley
3 tablespoons plain low-fat yogurt
3 tablespoons orange juice
2 tablespoons lime juice
2 tablespoons white wine vinegar
2 tablespoons water
1 tablespoon sugar
1 teaspoon chili powder
½ teaspoon onion powder
½ teaspoon ground cumin

Combine all ingredients in small jar with tight-fitting lid; shake well. Refrigerate until ready to use; shake before using. *Makes about ¾ cup*

Greek Pasta and Vegetable Salad

⅔ cup uncooked corkscrew macaroni
⅓ cup lime juice
2 tablespoons honey
1 tablespoon olive oil
1 clove garlic, finely chopped
4 cups washed and torn spinach leaves
1 cup sliced cucumber
½ cup thinly sliced carrot
¼ cup sliced green onions
2 tablespoons crumbled feta cheese
2 tablespoons sliced ripe olives

1. Prepare pasta according to package directions, omitting salt. Drain and rinse well under cold water until pasta is cool.

2. Blend lime juice, honey, oil and garlic in large bowl. Stir in pasta. Cover; marinate in refrigerator 2 to 24 hours.

3. Combine spinach, cucumber, carrot, onions, cheese and olives in large bowl. Add pasta mixture to salad; toss to combine. *Makes 4 servings*

NUTRIENTS PER SERVING:

Calories	188	Dietary Fiber	2 g
% calories from fat	28	Protein	5 g
Total Fat	6 g	Calcium	94 mg
Saturated Fat	1 g	Iron	3 mg
Cholesterol	3 mg	Vitamin A	794 RE
Sodium	230 mg	Vitamin C	27 mg
Carbohydrate	30 g		

Dietary Exchanges per Serving: 1 Starch/Bread, 2 Vegetable, 1 Fat

Scandinavian Beef & Vegetable Soup

1 tablespoon reduced-calorie margarine
¾ pound beef stew meat, cut into 1-inch pieces
4 cups fat-free reduced-sodium beef broth
⅔ cup coarsely chopped peeled potato
⅓ cup coarsely chopped peeled turnip
⅓ cup pearl onions
⅓ cup coarsely chopped carrot
1 bay leaf
½ teaspoon dried rosemary
¼ teaspoon ground allspice
⅛ teaspoon ground black pepper
4 teaspoons finely chopped fresh parsley

1. Melt margarine in large saucepan over medium heat. Add beef; cook and stir 5 minutes or until beef is browned. Add 4 cups water and beef broth. Bring to a boil over high heat. Reduce heat to medium-low. Simmer 1 hour or until beef is tender, stirring occasionally and skimming off any foam and fat that rises to surface.

2. Add potato, turnip, onions, carrot, bay leaf, rosemary, allspice and pepper to saucepan. Bring to a boil over high heat, stirring occasionally. Reduce heat to medium-low. Simmer 15 minutes or until vegetables are tender, stirring occasionally and skimming off any foam that rises to surface. Remove and discard bay leaf.

3. Top each serving evenly with parsley before serving. *Makes 4 servings*

NUTRIENTS PER SERVING:

Calories	186	Dietary Fiber	1 g
% calories from fat	30	Protein	20 g
Total Fat	6 g	Calcium	29 mg
Saturated Fat	2 g	Iron	2 mg
Cholesterol	50 mg	Vitamin A	298 RE
Sodium	141 mg	Vitamin C	8 mg
Carbohydrate	12 g		

Dietary Exchanges per Serving: ½ Starch/Bread, 2 Lean Meat, 1 Vegetable

Far East Tabbouleh

¾ cup uncooked bulgur
1¾ cups boiling water
2 tablespoons reduced-sodium teriyaki sauce
2 tablespoons lemon juice
1 tablespoon olive oil
¾ cup diced seeded cucumber
¾ cup diced seeded tomato
½ cup thinly sliced green onions
½ cup finely chopped fresh cilantro or parsley
1 tablespoon fresh ginger
1 clove garlic, crushed

1. Combine bulgur and boiling water in small bowl. Cover with plastic wrap; let stand 45 minutes or until bulgur is puffed, stirring occasionally. Drain in wire mesh sieve; discard liquid.

2. Combine bulgur, teriyaki sauce, lemon juice and oil in large bowl. Stir in cucumber, tomato, onions, cilantro, ginger and garlic until well blended. Cover; refrigerate 4 hours, stirring occasionally. Serve on fresh greens and garnish with sliced cucumber, tomato slices and fresh herbs, if desired.   *Makes 4 servings*

NUTRIENTS PER SERVING:

Calories	73	Dietary Fiber	3 g
% calories from fat	23	Protein	2 g
Total Fat	2 g	Calcium	16 mg
Saturated Fat	<1 g	Iron	1 mg
Cholesterol	0 mg	Vitamin A	51 RE
Sodium	156 mg	Vitamin C	9 mg
Carbohydrate	13 g		

Dietary Exchanges per Serving: ½ Starch/Bread, 1 Vegetable

Salmon Pasta Salad

1 cup cooked medium shells
1 can (6 ounces) canned red salmon, rinsed, drained
½ cup finely chopped celery
2 tablespoons finely chopped red bell pepper
2 tablespoons chopped fresh parsley
2 tablespoons fat-free mayonnaise
1 green onion, finely chopped
3 teaspoons lemon juice
2 teaspoons capers
⅛ teaspoon paprika

1. Combine pasta, salmon, celery, pepper, parsley, mayonnaise, onion, lemon juice, capers and paprika in medium bowl; blend well.

2. Cover; refrigerate 2 hours.   *Makes 2 servings*

NUTRIENTS PER SERVING:

Calories	262	Dietary Fiber	2 g
% calories from fat	32	Protein	18 g
Total Fat	9 g	Calcium	216 mg
Saturated Fat	2 g	Iron	2 mg
Cholesterol	21 mg	Vitamin A	153 RE
Sodium	627 mg	Vitamin C	44 mg
Carbohydrate	26 g		

Dietary Exchanges per Serving: 1½ Starch/Bread, 2 Lean Meat, 1 Vegetable, ½ Fat

Far East Tabbouleh

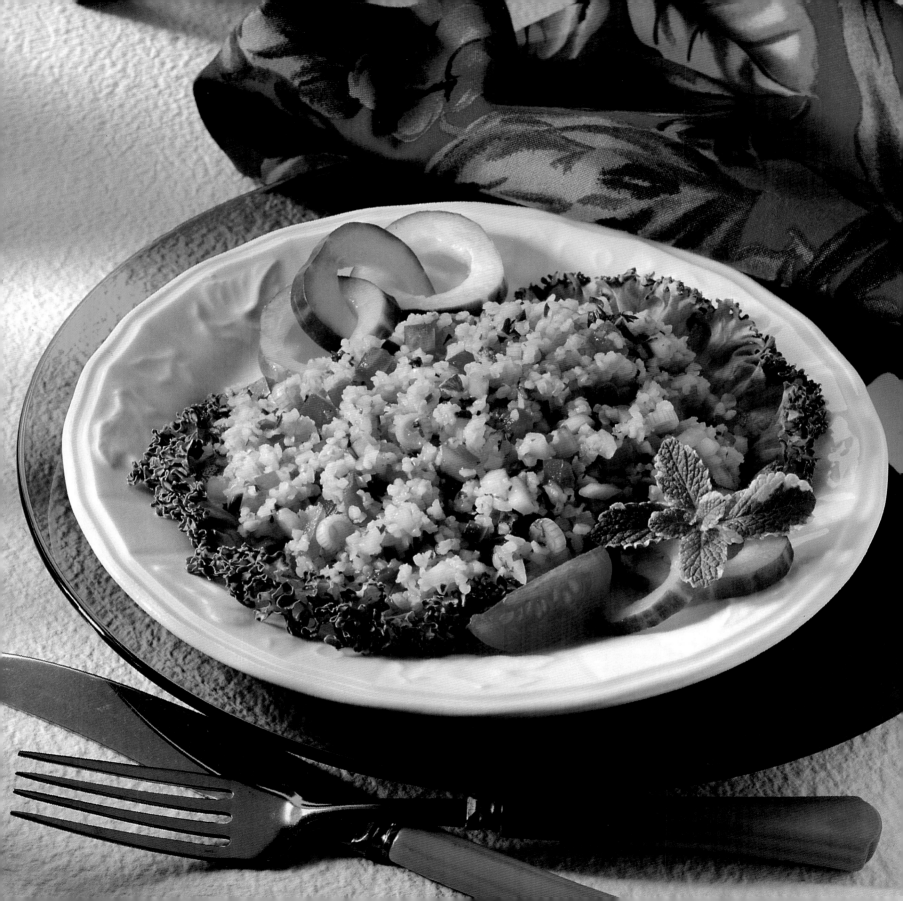

Pasta e Fagioli

2 tablespoons olive oil
1 cup chopped onion
3 cloves garlic, minced
2 cans (14½ ounces each) Italian-style stewed
    tomatoes
3 cups fat-free reduced-sodium chicken broth
1 can (about 15 ounces) cannellini beans (white
    kidney beans), undrained*
¼ cup chopped fresh Italian parsley
1 teaspoon dried basil leaves
¼ teaspoon ground black pepper
4 ounces uncooked small shell pasta

*One can (about 15 ounces) Great Northern beans, undrained,
may be substituted for cannellini beans.

1. Heat oil in 4-quart Dutch oven over medium heat
until hot; add onion and garlic. Cook and stir 5
minutes or until onion is tender.

2. Stir tomatoes, chicken broth, beans, parsley, basil
and pepper into Dutch oven; bring to a boil over high
heat, stirring occasionally. Cover; reduce heat to low.
Simmer 10 minutes.

3. Add pasta to Dutch oven. Cover; simmer 10 to 12
minutes or until pasta is just tender. Serve
immediately. Garnish as desired. *Makes 8 servings*

NUTRIENTS PER SERVING:

Calories	217	Dietary Fiber	6 g
% calories from fat	23	Protein	12 g
Total Fat	6 g	Calcium	65 mg
Saturated Fat	1 g	Iron	2 mg
Cholesterol	0 mg	Vitamin A	93 RE
Sodium	661 mg	Vitamin C	24 mg
Carbohydrate	37 g		

Dietary Exchanges per Serving: 2 Starch/Bread,
1 Vegetable, 1 Fat

Mexicali Bean & Cheese Salad

1 teaspoon vegetable oil
1 clove garlic, finely chopped
¼ cup finely chopped red onion
1½ teaspoons chili powder
¼ teaspoon ground cumin
⅛ teaspoon crushed red pepper
1 boneless skinless chicken breast (about
    6 ounces), cooked, shredded
1 cup frozen whole kernel corn, thawed
⅓ cup rinsed, drained canned pinto beans
⅓ cup rinsed, drained canned kidney beans
½ cup chopped seeded tomato
2 tablespoons drained canned diced mild green
    chilies
1 green onion, finely chopped
1 teaspoon lime juice
2 ounces reduced-fat Monterey Jack cheese,
    cut into ⅓-inch cubes

1. Heat oil in medium nonstick skillet over medium
heat until hot. Add garlic. Cook and stir 1 minute.
Add red onion, chili powder, cumin and red pepper.
Cook and stir 3 minutes. Add chicken, corn and
beans. Cook 5 minutes or until heated through,
stirring occasionally.

2. Combine bean mixture, tomato, chilies, green
onion and lime juice in medium serving bowl; toss to
combine. Add cheese; toss to combine. Refrigerate 2
hours before serving. *Makes 2 servings*

NUTRIENTS PER SERVING:

Calories	336	Dietary Fiber	6 g
% calories from fat	25	Protein	36 g
Total Fat	10 g	Calcium	310 mg
Saturated Fat	4 g	Iron	3 mg
Cholesterol	72 mg	Vitamin A	189 RE
Sodium	606 mg	Vitamin C	41 mg
Carbohydrate	36 g		

Dietary Exchanges per Serving: 2½ Starch/Bread,
3 Lean Meat, 1 Vegetable

Pasta e Fagioli

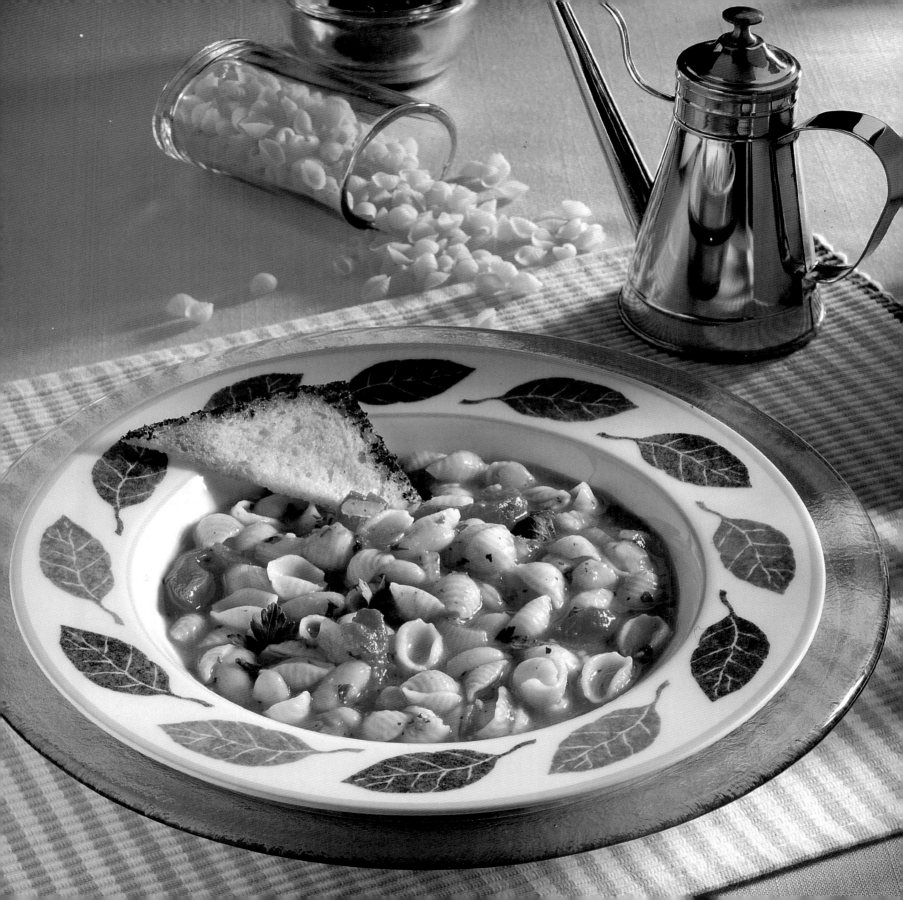

Roasted Winter Vegetable Soup

1 small *or* ½ medium acorn squash, halved
2 medium tomatoes
1 medium onion, unpeeled
1 green bell pepper, halved
1 red bell pepper, halved
2 small red potatoes
3 cloves garlic, unpeeled
1½ cups tomato juice
4 teaspoons vegetable oil
1 tablespoon red wine vinegar
¼ teaspoon ground black pepper
¾ cup chopped fresh cilantro
4 tablespoons nonfat sour cream

1. Preheat oven to 400°F. Spray baking sheet with nonstick cooking spray. Place acorn squash, tomatoes, onion, bell peppers, potatoes and garlic on baking sheet. Bake 40 minutes, removing garlic and tomatoes after 10 minutes. Let stand 15 minutes or until cool enough to handle.

2. Peel vegetables and garlic; discard skins. Coarsely chop vegetables. Combine half of chopped vegetables, tomato juice, ½ cup water, oil and vinegar in food processor or blender; process until smooth.

3. Combine puréed vegetables, remaining chopped vegetables and black pepper in large saucepan. Bring to a simmer over medium-high heat. Simmer 5 minutes or until heated through, stirring constantly. Top servings evenly with cilantro and sour cream.

Makes 4 servings

NUTRIENTS PER SERVING:

Calories	193	Dietary Fiber	5 g
% calories from fat	22	Protein	5 g
Total Fat	5 g	Calcium	84 mg
Saturated Fat	<1 g	Iron	2 mg
Cholesterol	0 mg	Vitamin A	330 RE
Sodium	345 mg	Vitamin C	92 mg
Carbohydrate	36 g		

Dietary Exchanges per Serving: 1½ Starch/Bread, 2 Vegetable, 1 Fat

Sunburst Chicken Salad

1 tablespoon fat-free mayonnaise
1 tablespoon nonfat sour cream
2 teaspoons frozen orange juice concentrate, thawed
¼ teaspoon grated orange peel
1 boneless skinless chicken breast, cooked, chopped
1 large kiwi, thinly sliced
⅓ cup mandarin oranges
¼ cup finely chopped celery
4 lettuce leaves, washed
2 tablespoons coarsely chopped cashews

1. Blend mayonnaise, sour cream, concentrate and orange peel in small bowl.

2. Add chicken, kiwi, oranges and celery; toss to coat. Cover; refrigerate 2 hours. Serve on lettuce leaves. Top with cashews before serving. *Makes 2 servings*

NUTRIENTS PER SERVING:

Calories	195	Dietary Fiber	2 g
% calories from fat	29	Protein	18 g
Total Fat	6 g	Calcium	55 mg
Saturated Fat	1 g	Iron	1 mg
Cholesterol	39 mg	Vitamin A	68 RE
Sodium	431 mg	Vitamin C	61 mg
Carbohydrate	18 g		

Dietary Exchanges per Serving: 2 Lean Meat, 1 Fruit, ½ Fat

Sunburst Chicken Salad

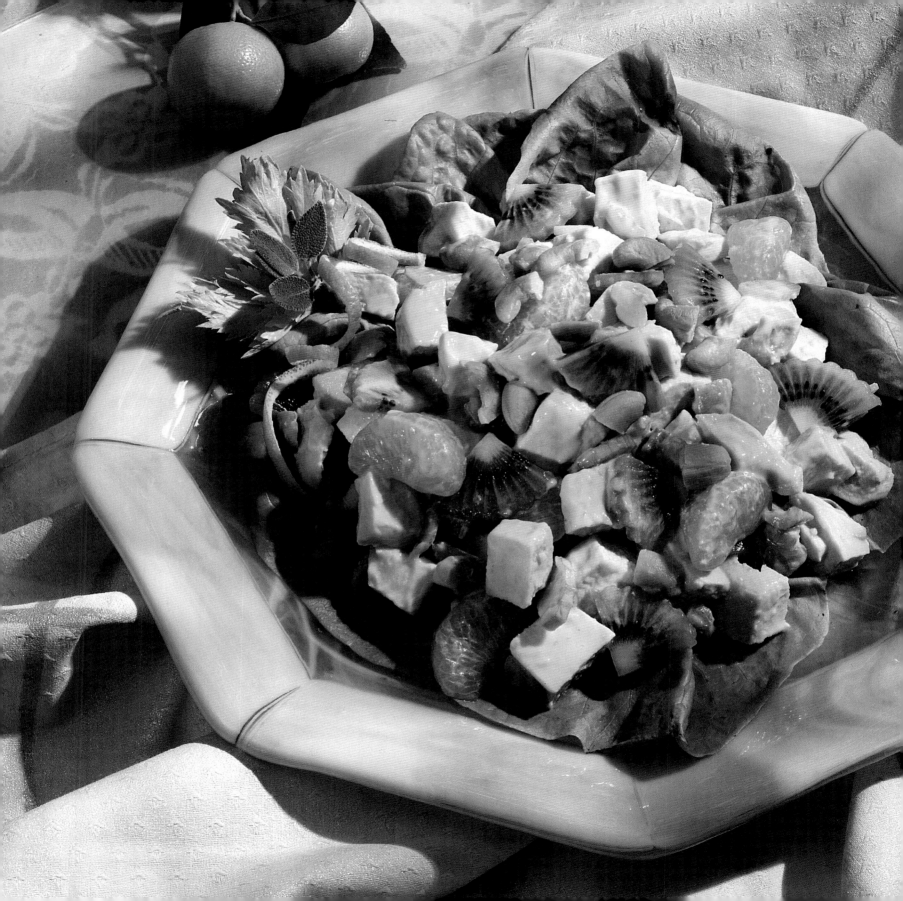

Layered Mexican Salad

**1 small head romaine lettuce, washed, cored
Salsa Cruda (recipe follows)
1 can (15 ounces) black turtle beans, rinsed, drained
1 cup frozen whole kernel corn, thawed, drained
1 large cucumber, peeled
1 can (2¼ ounces) sliced ripe olives, drained
1 large lemon
¾ cup nonfat mayonnaise
3 tablespoons plain nonfat yogurt
2 to 3 cloves garlic, minced
½ cup (2 ounces) shredded low-fat Cheddar cheese
1 green onion, thinly sliced**

1. Layer romaine leaves and slice crosswise into ½-inch strips. Place half of lettuce in large serving bowl. Layer Salsa Cruda, beans and corn over lettuce.

2. Halve cucumber lengthwise; scoop out and discard seeds. Slice thinly. Place cucumber over corn, sprinkle with olives and top with remaining lettuce.

3. Grate lemon peel; blend with mayonnaise, yogurt and garlic. Juice lemon; stir 3 to 4 tablespoons juice into dressing. Spread dressing evenly over top of salad. Sprinkle with cheese and green onion. Cover salad and refrigerate 2 hours or up to 1 day.

Makes 12 servings

NUTRIENTS PER SERVING:

Calories	117	Dietary Fiber	3 g
% calories from fat	22	Protein	6 g
Total Fat	3 g	Calcium	77 mg
Saturated Fat	1 g	Iron	2 mg
Cholesterol	3 mg	Vitamin A	121 RE
Sodium	349 mg	Vitamin C	18 mg
Carbohydrate	19 g		

Dietary Exchanges per Serving: 1 Starch/Bread, 1 Vegetable, 1 Fat

Salsa Cruda

**1 cup chopped seeded tomato
2 tablespoons finely chopped onion
2 tablespoons finely chopped fresh cilantro (optional)
2 tablespoons lime juice
½ jalapeño pepper, seeded, finely chopped*
1 clove garlic, minced**

*Jalapeño peppers can sting and irritate the skin. Wear rubber gloves when handling peppers and do not touch eyes.

Combine tomato, onion, cilantro, if desired, lime juice, pepper and garlic in small bowl; blend well.

Makes 4 servings

Health Note: Nearly 50 percent of adults with high blood pressure do not experience a reduction in elevated levels when the amount of sodium in their diet is reduced. Blood pressure levels are much more responsive to a calcium-rich meal plan. Researchers now believe that good-for-your-bones calcium plays a major role in the maintenance of near normal blood pressure levels.

Layered Mexican Salad

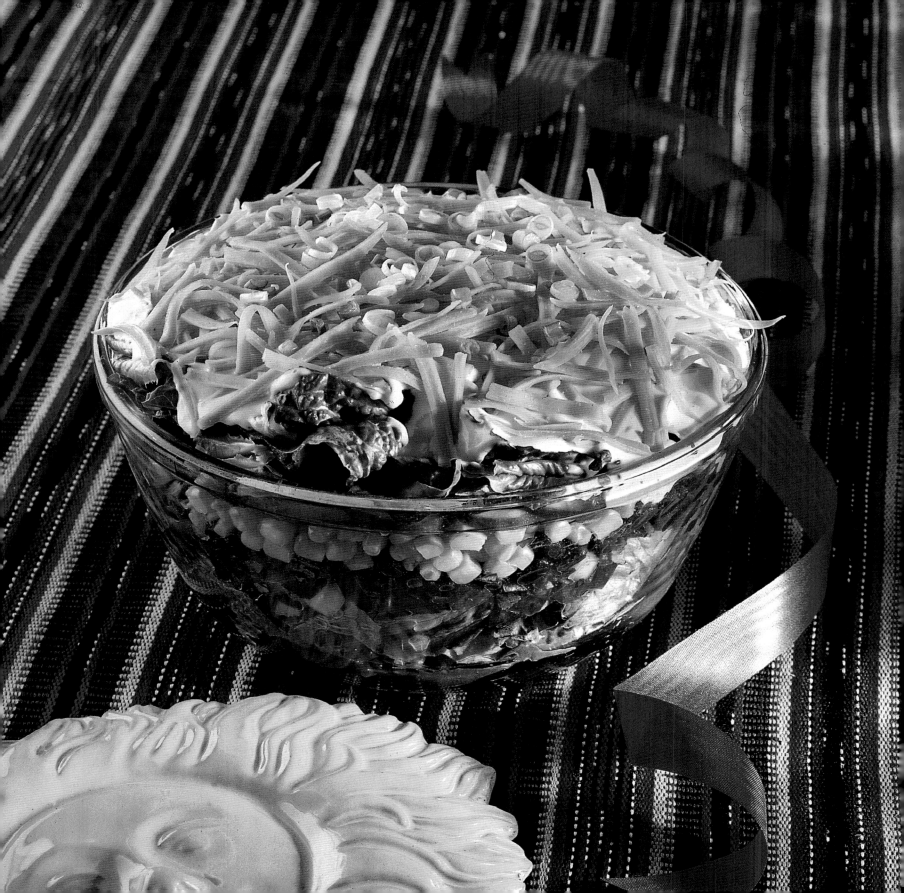

DELICIOUS DINNERS

Transform ho-hum meals into dynamite dinners with these mouthwatering entrées prepared with delicious Mexican, Oriental and Italian fixings.

Linguine with Pesto-Marinara Clam Sauce

1 teaspoon vegetable oil
¼ cup chopped shallots
3 cloves garlic, finely chopped
2 cans (6 ounces each) minced clams
1⅓ cups Marinara Sauce (page 56)
2 tablespoons prepared pesto sauce
¼ teaspoon crushed red pepper
8 ounces uncooked linguine
¼ cup chopped fresh parsley

1. Heat oil in large nonstick saucepan over medium heat until hot. Add shallots and garlic. Cook, covered, 2 minutes.

2. Drain clams; reserve ½ cup juice. Add clams, reserved juice, Marinara Sauce, pesto and red pepper to saucepan. Cook 10 minutes, stirring occasionally.

3. Prepare linguine according to package directions, omitting salt. Drain. Spoon sauce evenly over each serving; top with parsley. Garnish with lemon slices and additional parsley, if desired.

Makes 4 servings

NUTRIENTS PER SERVING:

Calories	398	Dietary Fiber	4 g
% calories from fat	13	Protein	32 g
Total Fat	6 g	Calcium	146 mg
Saturated Fat	1 g	Iron	27 mg
Cholesterol	58 mg	Vitamin A	407 RE
Sodium	293 mg	Vitamin C	34 mg
Carbohydrate	54 g		

Dietary Exchanges per Serving: 2½ Starch/Bread, 3 Lean Meat, 2½ Vegetable

Linguine with Pesto-Marinara Clam Sauce

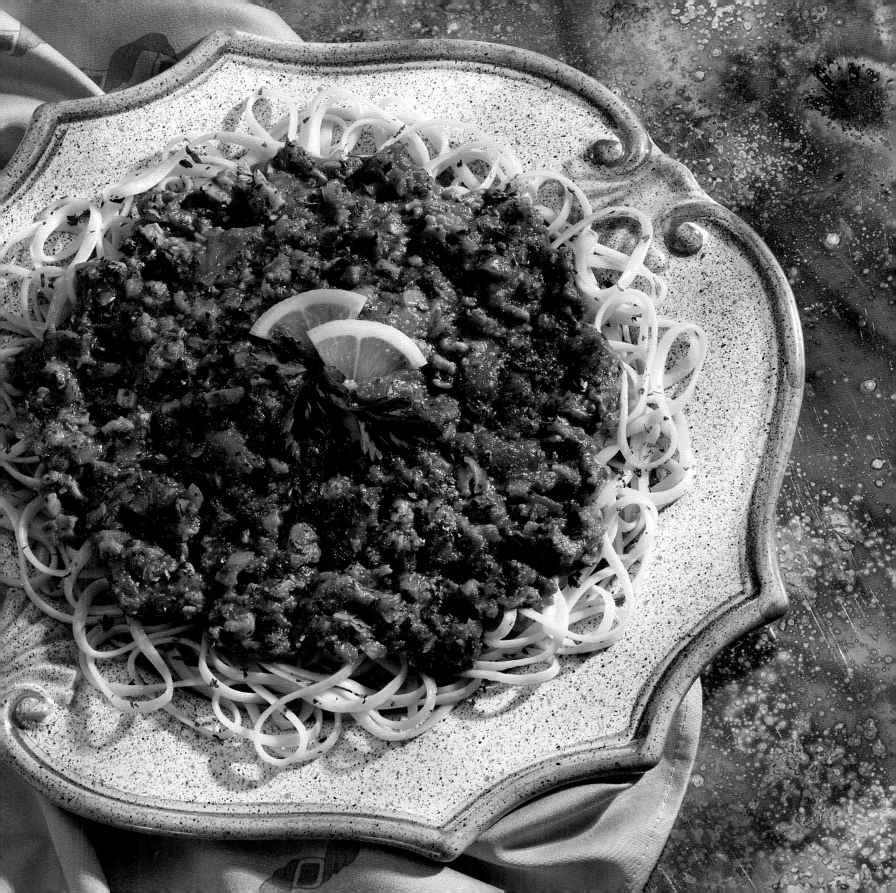

Crispy Baked Chicken

4 skinless chicken breast halves (1½ pounds)
2 tablespoons plus 1½ teaspoons Dijon mustard, divided
1 cup fresh whole wheat bread crumbs
½ teaspoon dried marjoram leaves
½ teaspoon dried thyme leaves
¼ teaspoon salt
¼ teaspoon dried sage leaves
¼ teaspoon ground black pepper
Nonstick cooking spray
1 small red bell pepper, sliced
2 cloves garlic, minced
2 cups broccoli flowerets, cooked crisp-tender
1 to 2 tablespoons lemon juice

1. Preheat oven to 375°F. Brush tops of chicken breasts with 2 tablespoons mustard. Combine bread crumbs, marjoram, thyme, salt, sage and black pepper in small bowl. Pat mixture evenly onto mustard. Arrange chicken breasts in single layer in 13×9-inch baking pan. Bake, uncovered, 40 minutes or until chicken is no longer pink in center.

2. Generously spray medium skillet with cooking spray; heat over medium heat until hot. Add bell pepper and garlic; cook and stir 5 minutes or until tender. Add broccoli and lemon juice; cook and stir 2 to 3 minutes or until heated through. Serve chicken with broccoli mixture. *Makes 4 servings*

NUTRIENTS PER SERVING:

Calories	196	Dietary Fiber	3 g
% calories from fat	18	Protein	29 g
Total Fat	4 g	Calcium	66 mg
Saturated Fat	1 g	Iron	2 mg
Cholesterol	69 mg	Vitamin A	86 RE
Sodium	412 mg	Vitamin C	62 mg
Carbohydrate	11 g		

Dietary Exchanges per Serving: ½ Starch/Bread, 2½ Lean Meat, 1 Vegetable

Fragrant Beef with Garlic Sauce

⅓ cup teriyaki sauce
1 boneless beef top sirloin steak, cut 1 inch thick (about 1¼ pounds)
10 large cloves garlic, peeled
½ cup fat-free reduced-sodium beef broth
4 cups hot cooked white rice

1. Place teriyaki sauce in large resealable plastic food storage bag; add beef. Seal bag; turn to coat. Marinate in refrigerator 30 minutes or up to 4 hours, turning occasionally.

2. Preheat broiler. Combine garlic and beef broth in small saucepan; bring to a boil over high heat. Reduce heat to medium; simmer 5 minutes. Cover; simmer 8 to 9 minutes until garlic is softened. Transfer to food processor or blender; process until smooth.

3. Meanwhile, drain beef; reserve marinade. Spray rack of broiler pan with nonstick cooking spray. Place beef on rack; brush with half of reserved marinade. Broil 4 inches from heat 10 minutes or until desired doneness, turning occasionally and basting with remaining marinade. (Do not brush with marinade during last 5 minutes of cooking.)

4. Thinly slice beef. Spoon garlic sauce over beef and rice. *Makes 4 servings*

NUTRIENTS PER SERVING:

Calories	411	Dietary Fiber	1 g
% calories from fat	29	Protein	37 g
Total Fat	13 g	Calcium	36 mg
Saturated Fat	5 g	Iron	4 mg
Cholesterol	95 mg	Vitamin A	6 RE
Sodium	480 mg	Vitamin C	3 mg
Carbohydrate	48 g		

Dietary Exchanges per Serving: 2½ Starch/Bread, 3½ Lean Meat

Crispy Baked Chicken

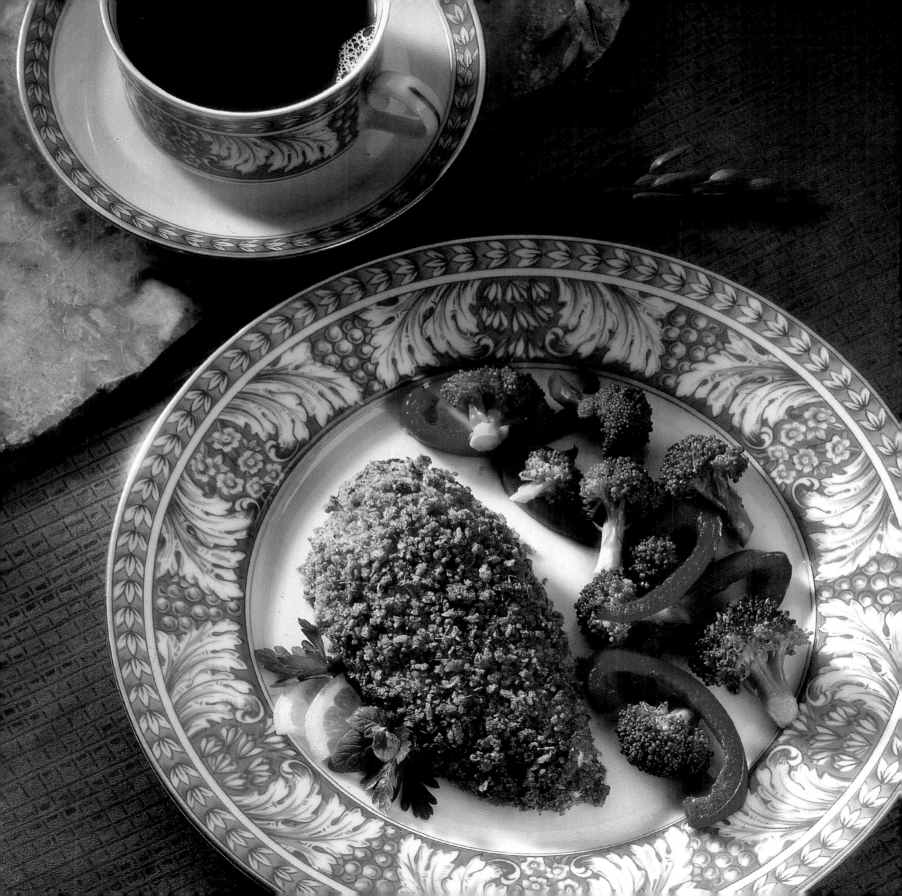

Turkey Vegetable Chili Mac

¾ pound ground turkey breast
½ cup chopped onion
2 cloves garlic, minced
1 can (about 15 ounces) black beans, rinsed and drained
1 can (14½ ounces) Mexican-style stewed tomatoes
1 can (14½ ounces) no-salt-added diced tomatoes
1 cup frozen whole kernel corn
1 teaspoon Mexican seasoning
½ cup uncooked elbow macaroni
⅓ cup reduced-fat sour cream

1. Spray large nonstick saucepan or Dutch oven with nonstick cooking spray. Add turkey, onion and garlic; cook 5 minutes or until turkey is no longer pink, stirring to crumble.

2. Add beans, tomatoes, corn and Mexican seasoning to saucepan; bring to a boil over high heat. Cover; reduce heat to low. Simmer 15 minutes, stirring occasionally.

3. Meanwhile, cook pasta according to package directions, omitting salt; drain. Stir into saucepan. Simmer 2 to 3 minutes or until heated through.

4. Top each serving with dollop of sour cream. Garnish as desired. *Makes 6 servings*

NUTRIENTS PER SERVING:

Calories	236	Dietary Fiber	6 g
% calories from fat	21	Protein	17 g
Total Fat	6 g	Calcium	73 mg
Saturated Fat	1 g	Iron	2 mg
Cholesterol	25 mg	Vitamin A	151 RE
Sodium	445 mg	Vitamin C	22 mg
Carbohydrate	34 g		

Dietary Exchanges per Serving: 1½ Starch/Bread, 1 Lean Meat, 2 Vegetable, ½ Fat

Pork with Couscous & Root Vegetables

1 teaspoon vegetable oil
½ pound pork tenderloin, thinly sliced
2 sweet potatoes, peeled, chopped
2 medium turnips, peeled, chopped
1 carrot, sliced
3 cloves garlic, finely chopped
1 can (about 15 ounces) garbanzo beans (chick-peas), rinsed and drained
1 cup fat-free reduced-sodium vegetable broth
½ cup pitted prunes, cut into thirds
1 teaspoon ground cumin
½ teaspoon ground cinnamon
¼ teaspoon ground allspice
¼ teaspoon ground nutmeg
¼ teaspoon ground black pepper
1 cup uncooked quick-cooking couscous, cooked
2 tablespoons dried currants

1. Heat oil in large nonstick skillet over medium-high heat until hot. Add pork, sweet potatoes, turnips, carrot and garlic. Cook and stir 5 minutes. Stir in beans, vegetable broth, prunes, cumin, cinnamon, allspice, nutmeg and pepper. Cover; bring to a boil over high heat. Reduce heat to medium-low. Simmer 30 minutes.

2. Serve pork and vegetables on couscous. Top servings evenly with currants. *Makes 4 servings*

NUTRIENTS PER SERVING:

Calories	508	Dietary Fiber	17 g
% calories from fat	11	Protein	26 g
Total Fat	6 g	Calcium	117 mg
Saturated Fat	1 g	Iron	5 mg
Cholesterol	30 mg	Vitamin A	1,793 RE
Sodium	500 mg	Vitamin C	28 mg
Carbohydrate	88 g		

Dietary Exchanges per Serving: 4 Starch/Bread, 2 Lean Meat, 1 Fruit, 2 Vegetable

Turkey Vegetable Chili Mac

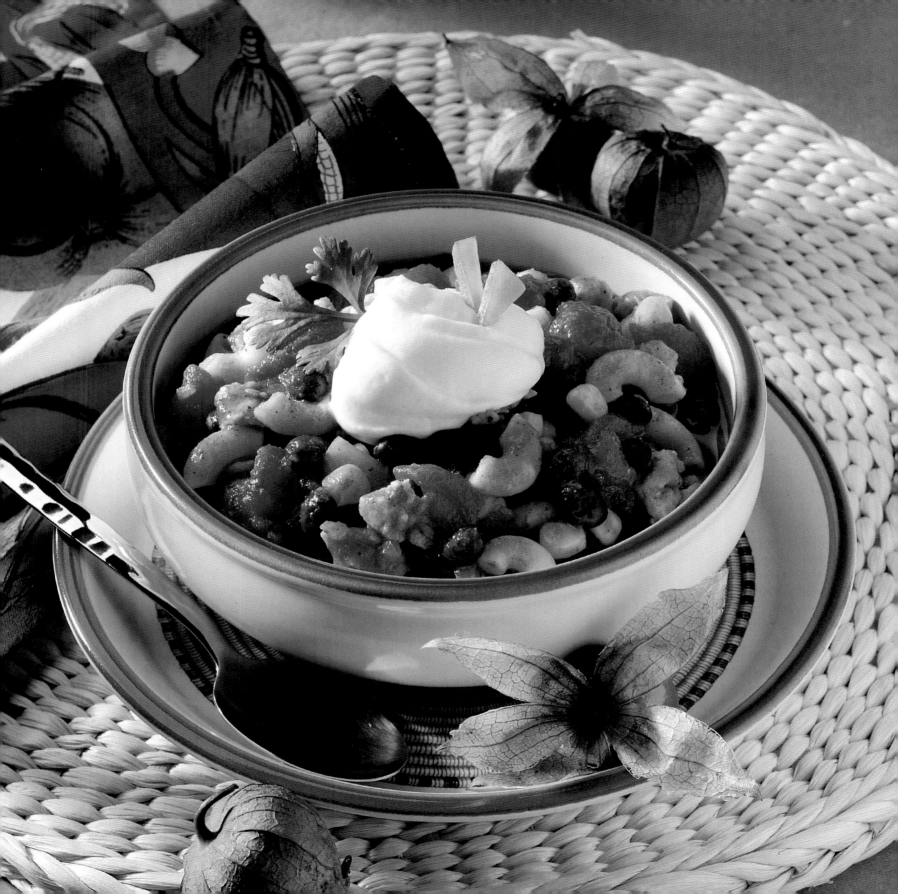

Rio Grande Bean Enchiladas

3 teaspoons olive oil, divided
2 cups chopped onions, divided
1 can (14½ ounces) crushed tomatoes
1 can (6 ounces) tomato paste
2 tablespoons chili powder
1 tablespoon prepared green salsa
2 teaspoons ground cumin, divided
1 teaspoon sugar
⅛ teaspoon ground black pepper
2 cloves garlic, finely chopped
1 can (about 15 ounces) black beans, rinsed, drained, mashed
1 cup plain nonfat yogurt
8 (6-inch) corn tortillas

1. Heat 2 teaspoons oil in large saucepan over medium-high heat. Add 1 cup onions. Cook and stir 5 minutes. Stir in tomatoes, tomato paste, chili powder, salsa, 1 teaspoon cumin, sugar and pepper. Reduce heat to medium-low. Simmer 30 minutes.

2. Heat remaining 1 teaspoon oil in large skillet over medium-high heat until hot. Add remaining 1 cup onions, 1 teaspoon cumin and garlic. Cook and stir 5 minutes or until onions are tender. Stir in beans. Cook 5 minutes or until heated through, stirring occasionally. Remove skillet from heat. Stir in yogurt.

3. Preheat oven to 375°F. Spoon bean mixture evenly down centers of tortillas. Roll up tortillas; place in medium baking dish. Top with sauce. Bake 20 minutes. Serve with dollops of nonfat sour cream and cilantro, if desired. Garnish with cilantro and red pepper strips, if desired. *Makes 4 servings*

NUTRIENTS PER SERVING:

Calories	365	Dietary Fiber	11 g
% calories from fat	17	Protein	19 g
Total Fat	7 g	Calcium	282 mg
Saturated Fat	1 g	Iron	4 mg
Cholesterol	1 mg	Vitamin A	315 RE
Sodium	1,050 mg	Vitamin C	44 mg
Carbohydrate	69 g		

Dietary Exchanges per Serving: 3 Starch/Bread, 4 Vegetable, 1½ Fat

Pasta Primavera

4 ounces uncooked spinach fettuccine
1 cup plain nonfat yogurt
¼ cup packed fresh parsley
¼ cup packed fresh chives
½ teaspoon salt
¼ teaspoon ground black pepper
1 teaspoon margarine
1 teaspoon vegetable oil
½ pound fresh or thawed frozen asparagus, cut diagonally into ½-inch pieces
1 cup thinly sliced carrots
1 cup thawed frozen green peas
¾ cup thawed frozen cut green beans
3 cloves garlic, finely chopped
2 tablespoons grated Parmesan cheese

1. Cook fettuccine according to package directions, omitting salt. Drain fettuccine. Set aside.

2. In food processor or blender combine yogurt, parsley, chives, salt and pepper; process until smooth.

3. Heat margarine and oil in medium saucepan over medium heat until hot. Add asparagus, carrots, peas, beans and garlic. Cook and stir 8 minutes or until vegetables are tender. Stir in pasta and yogurt mixture. Cook 3 minutes or until heated through, stirring occasionally. Sprinkle cheese evenly over each serving. Serve immediately. *Makes 4 servings*

NUTRIENTS PER SERVING:

Calories	339	Dietary Fiber	3 g
% calories from fat	13	Protein	16 g
Total Fat	5 g	Calcium	253 mg
Saturated Fat	2 g	Iron	3 mg
Cholesterol	6 mg	Vitamin A	893 RE
Sodium	422 mg	Vitamin C	42 mg
Carbohydrate	58 g		

Dietary Exchanges per Serving: 3 Starch/Bread, ½ Milk, 1½ Vegetable, ½ Fat

Rio Grande Bean Enchiladas

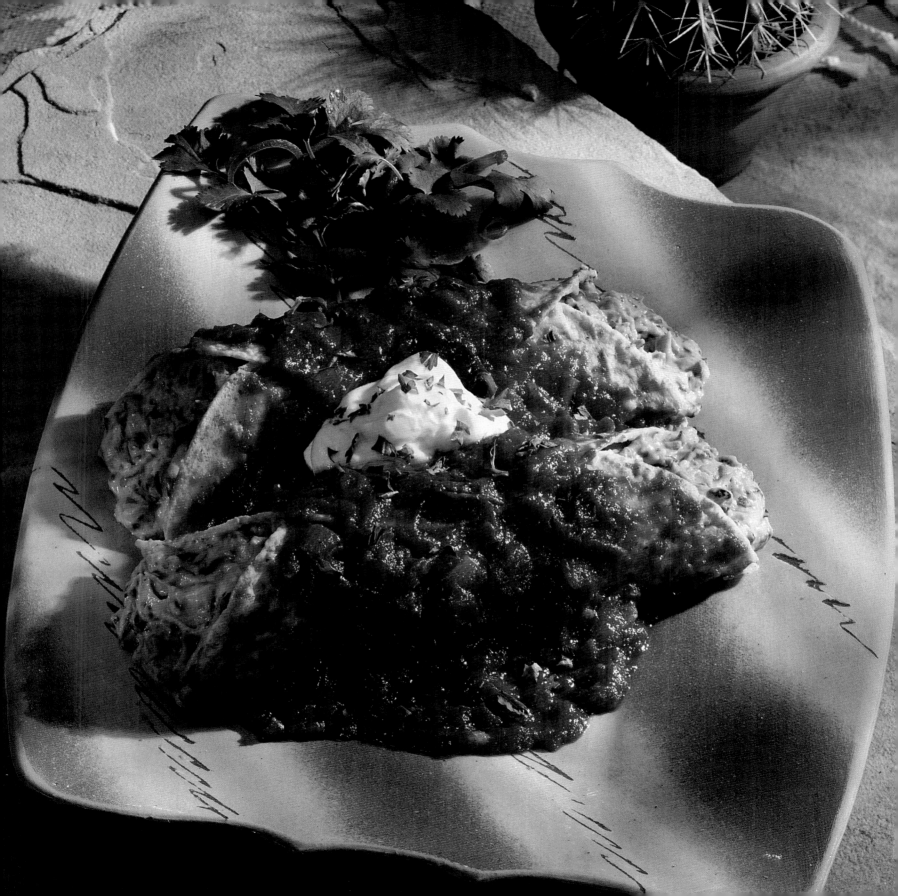

Mediterranean Chicken Kabobs

2 pounds boneless skinless chicken breasts or chicken tenders, cut into 1-inch pieces
1 small eggplant, peeled, cut into 1-inch pieces
1 medium zucchini, cut crosswise into ½-inch slices
2 medium onions, each cut into 8 wedges
16 medium mushrooms, stems removed
16 cherry tomatoes
1 cup fat-free reduced-sodium chicken broth
⅔ cup balsamic vinegar
3 tablespoons olive oil or vegetable oil
2 tablespoons dried mint leaves
4 teaspoons dried basil leaves
1 tablespoon dried oregano leaves
2 teaspoons grated lemon peel
Chopped fresh parsley (optional)
4 cups hot cooked couscous

1. Alternately thread chicken and vegetables onto 16 metal skewers; place in large glass baking dish. Blend chicken broth, vinegar, oil, mint, basil and oregano in small bowl. Pour over kabobs; turn to coat. Cover; marinate in refrigerator 2 hours, turning occasionally.

2. Preheat broiler. Spray rack of broiler pan with nonstick cooking spray. Place kabobs on rack. Broil, 6 inches from heat, 10 to 15 minutes or until chicken is no longer pink in center, turning occasionally. Stir lemon peel and parsley, if desired, into couscous; serve with kabobs. *Makes 8 servings*

NUTRIENTS PER SERVING:

Calories	293	Dietary Fiber	7 g
% calories from fat	23	Protein	22 g
Total Fat	8 g	Calcium	56 mg
Saturated Fat	1 g	Iron	3 mg
Cholesterol	46 mg	Vitamin A	49 RE
Sodium	60 mg	Vitamin C	16 mg
Carbohydrate	34 g		

Dietary Exchanges per Serving: 1½ Starch/Bread, 2 Lean Meat, 2 Vegetable, ½ Fat

Shrimp Tostadas

Nonstick cooking spray
1 can (about 15 ounces) kidney beans, rinsed, drained, mashed
1 tablespoon chili powder
2 teaspoons ground cumin
½ teaspoon garlic powder
4 (6-inch) flour tortillas
3 cups shredded lettuce leaves
8 ounces cooked medium shrimp
2 cups Spicy Salsa, (page 20)
4 tablespoons plain nonfat yogurt

1. Preheat oven to 375°F.

2. Spray medium nonstick skillet with cooking spray. Heat over medium heat until hot. Add beans, chili powder, cumin and garlic powder. Cook and stir 5 minutes or until heated through. Reduce heat to low.

3. Place tortillas on baking sheet. Bake 3 to 4 minutes or until tortillas are crisp.

4. Spread bean mixture evenly over tortillas. Top tortillas evenly with lettuce and shrimp. Spoon salsa evenly over tortillas; top with dollops of yogurt. Serve immediately. *Makes 4 servings*

NUTRIENTS PER SERVING:

Calories	303	Dietary Fiber	10 g
% calories from fat	11	Protein	26 g
Total Fat	4 g	Calcium	88 mg
Saturated Fat	1 g	Iron	3 mg
Cholesterol	111 mg	Vitamin A	260 RE
Sodium	392 mg	Vitamin C	27 mg
Carbohydrate	48 g		

Dietary Exchanges per Serving: 2½ Starch/Bread, 2 Lean Meat, 1 Vegetable

Mediterranean Chicken Kabobs

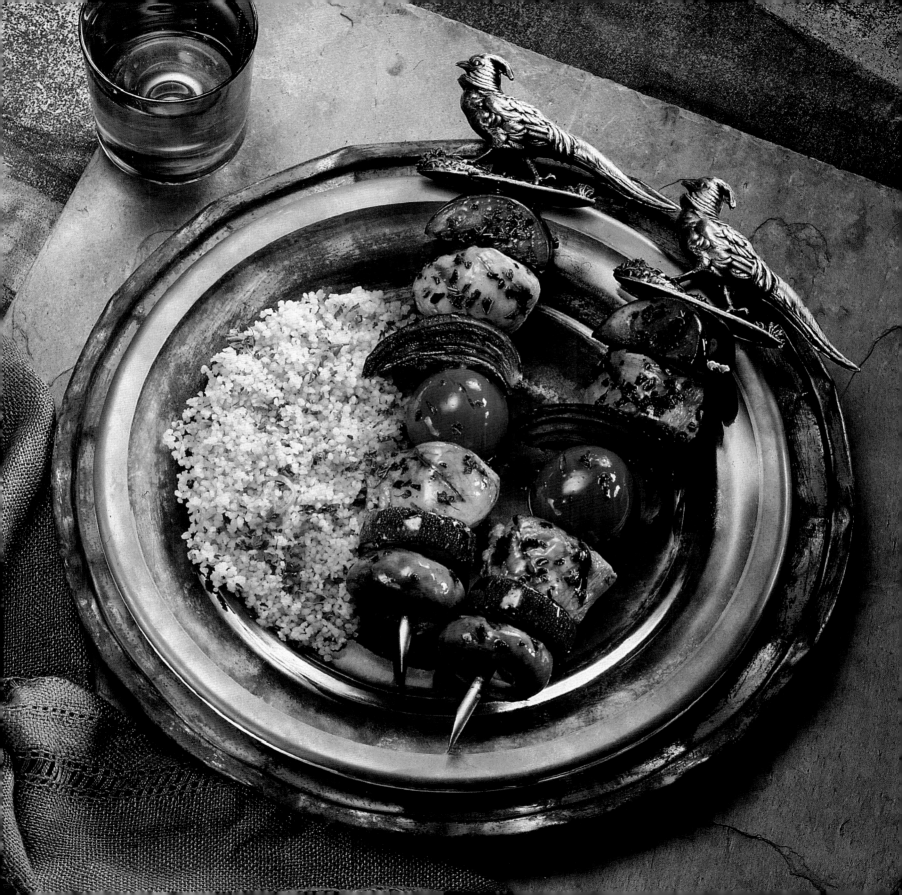

Hearty Cassoulet

1 tablespoon olive oil
1 large onion, finely chopped
4 boneless skinless chicken thighs (about
    1 pound), chopped
¼ pound smoked turkey sausage, finely
    chopped
3 cloves garlic, finely chopped
3 cans (about 15 ounces each) Great Northern
    beans, rinsed and drained
4 tablespoons tomato paste
1 teaspoon dried thyme leaves
½ teaspoon ground black pepper
½ cup bread crumbs
3 tablespoons finely chopped fresh parsley

1. Heat oil in ovenproof skillet over medium-high heat until hot. Add onion; cook and stir 5 minutes or until onion is tender. Add chicken, sausage and garlic; cook 5 minutes or until chicken and sausage are browned, stirring occasionally.

2. Add beans, ¼ cup water, tomato paste, thyme and pepper to skillet. Cover; reduce heat to medium-low. Simmer 15 minutes or until mixture is bubbly.

3. Preheat broiler. Combine bread crumbs and parsley in small bowl; sprinkle over top of cassoulet. Broil, 4 inches from heat, 3 minutes or until bread crumbs are lightly browned.

Makes 6 servings

NUTRIENTS PER SERVING:

Calories	432	Dietary Fiber	1 g
% calories from fat	18	Protein	31 g
Total Fat	9 g	Calcium	176 mg
Saturated Fat	2 g	Iron	6 mg
Cholesterol	45 mg	Vitamin A	44 RE
Sodium	365 mg	Vitamin C	12 mg
Carbohydrate	59 g		

Dietary Exchanges per Serving: 3½ Starch/Bread,
3 Lean Meat, 1 Vegetable

Spaghetti with Marinara Sauce

1 teaspoon olive oil
¾ cup chopped onion
3 cloves garlic, finely chopped
1 can (16 ounces) no-salt-added tomato sauce
1 can (6 ounces) tomato paste
2 bay leaves
1 teaspoon dried oregano
1 teaspoon dried basil
½ teaspoon dried marjoram
½ teaspoon honey
¼ teaspoon black pepper
8 ounces uncooked spaghetti

1. Heat oil in large saucepan. Add onion and garlic. Cook and stir 5 minutes or until onion is tender. Add 2 cups water, tomato sauce, tomato paste, bay leaves, oregano, basil, marjoram, honey and pepper. Bring to a boil, stirring occasionally. Reduce heat; simmer 1 hour, stirring occasionally. Remove and discard bay leaves.

2. Cook pasta according to package directions, omitting salt. Drain. Measure 2 cups sauce; reserve remaining sauce for another use. Serve sauce on pasta.

Makes 4 servings

NUTRIENTS PER SERVING:

Calories	289	Dietary Fiber	3 g
% calories from fat	<1	Protein	10 g
Total Fat	2 g	Calcium	41 mg
Saturated Fat	<1 g	Iron	4 mg
Cholesterol	0 mg	Vitamin A	126 RE
Sodium	213 mg	Vitamin C	20 mg
Carbohydrate	58 g		

Dietary Exchanges per Serving: 3 Starch/Bread,
2½ Vegetable

Hearty Cassoulet

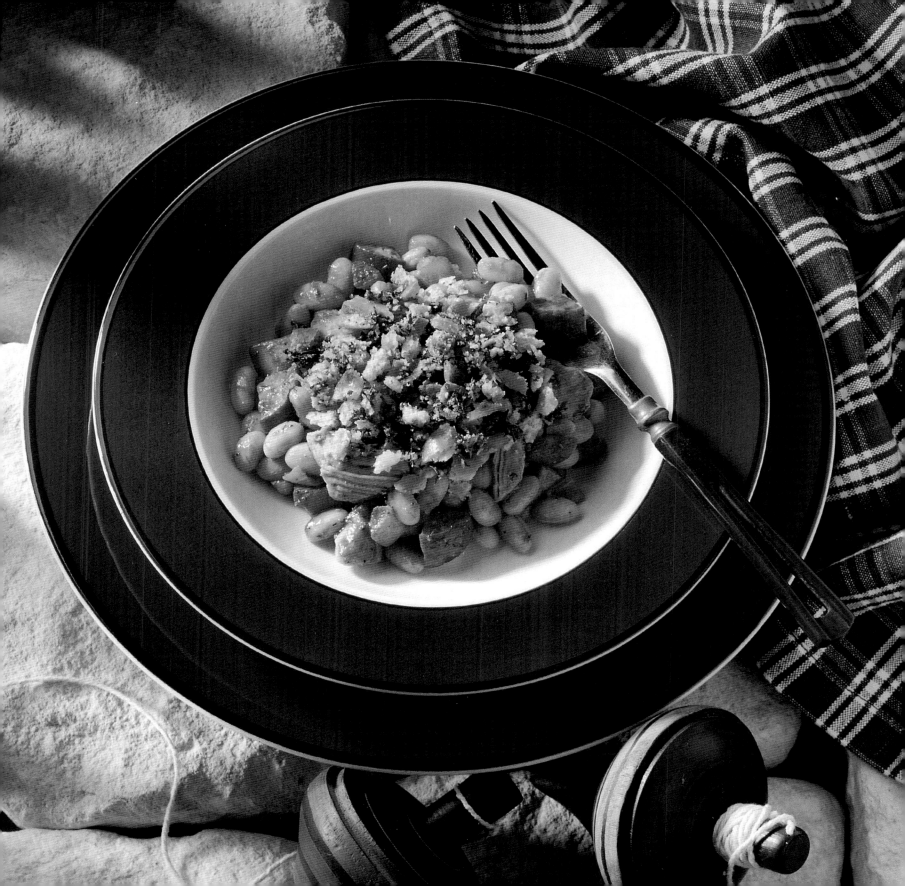

Lemon-Crusted Country Pie

½ cup plus 2 tablespoons all-purpose flour,
    divided
⅓ cup whole wheat flour
1 teaspoon grated lemon peel
2 tablespoons vegetable oil
3 to 4 tablespoons ice water
    Nonstick cooking spray
1 boneless skinless chicken breast, chopped
    (about 4 ounces)
1 cup chopped onion
1 cup chopped celery
1 cup sliced mushrooms
½ cup shredded carrot
1 tablespoon margarine
½ cup fat-free reduced-sodium chicken broth
½ cup skim milk
½ teaspoon salt
½ teaspoon dried rosemary
¼ teaspoon ground black pepper
1 cup frozen whole kernel corn
1 cup frozen green peas
⅓ cup fresh or dry whole wheat bread crumbs

1. Combine ½ cup all-purpose flour, whole wheat flour and lemon peel in medium bowl. Add oil; blend well. Add water, 1 tablespoon at a time, until soft dough forms. Flatten dough into disc; cover with plastic wrap. Refrigerate 30 minutes.

2. Place dough on lightly floured surface. Roll out dough into 10-inch circle, ⅛ inch thick. Ease dough into 9-inch pie plate. (If excess dough remains, reroll and cut out decorative shapes.)

3. Spray large skillet with cooking spray. Add chicken. Cook and stir 3 minutes. Add vegetables. Cook and stir 5 minutes or until chicken is no longer pink.

4. Preheat oven to 375°F. Melt margarine in medium saucepan over medium heat. Add remaining 2 tablespoons flour. Cook and stir 3 minutes. Gradually stir in chicken broth, milk, salt, rosemary and pepper.

5. Cook 6 minutes or until sauce thickens, stirring constantly. Stir in chicken mixture, corn, peas and bread crumbs. Remove saucepan from heat; let stand 15 minutes.

6. Spoon vegetable mixture into prepared crust. (Arrange cutouts over top of pie, if desired.) Brush with additional milk.

7. Bake 50 minutes or until filling is set. (If crust browns too much before filling sets, cover crust with aluminum foil.) *Makes 4 servings*

NUTRIENTS PER SERVING:

Calories	372	Dietary Fiber	6 g
% calories from fat	29	Protein	19 g
Total Fat	12 g	Calcium	97 mg
Saturated Fat	2 g	Iron	3 mg
Cholesterol	28 mg	Vitamin A	540 RE
Sodium	449 mg	Vitamin C	13 mg
Carbohydrate	47 g		

Dietary Exchanges per Serving: 2½ Starch/Bread,
1 Lean Meat, 2 Vegetable, 2 Fat

Lemon-Crusted Country Pie

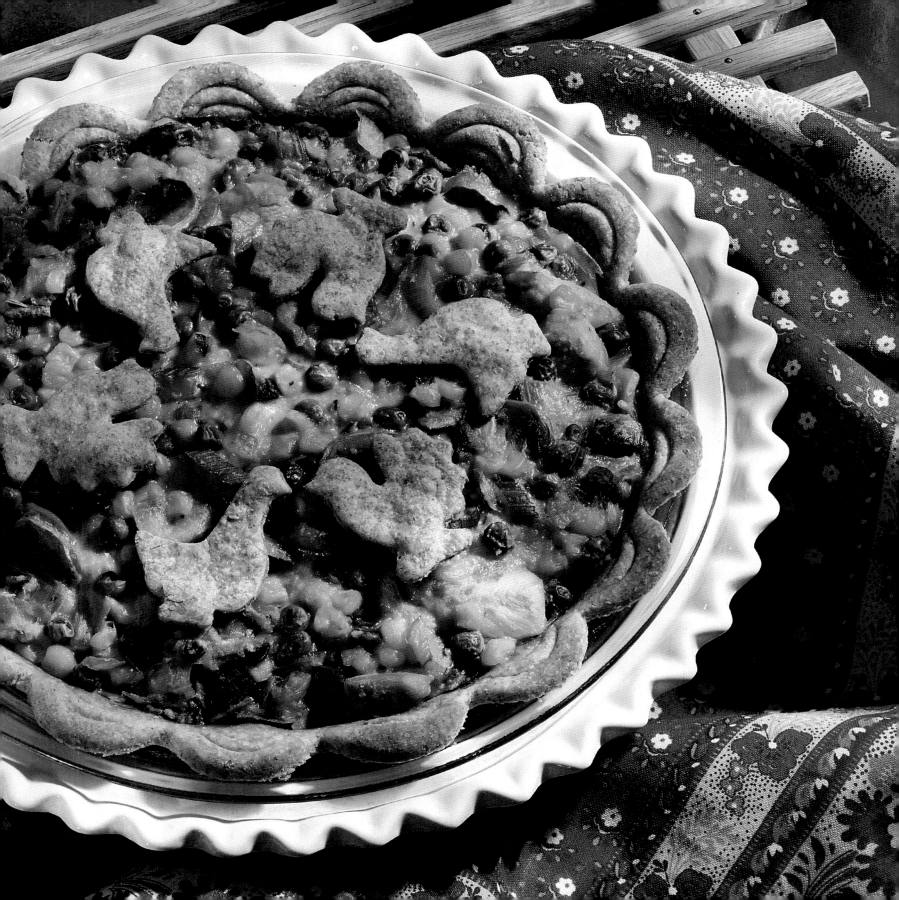

Pork with Sweet Hungarian Paprika

1 teaspoon olive oil, divided
1 onion, sliced
2 cloves garlic, finely chopped
1 tomato, chopped
1 red bell pepper, chopped
1 large Anaheim *or* 1 medium green bell pepper, chopped
1 can (10½ ounces) fat-free reduced-sodium chicken broth, divided
2 tablespoons sweet Hungarian paprika
12 ounces pork tenderloin
3 tablespoons all-purpose flour
⅓ cup low-fat sour cream
6 cups cooked enriched egg noodles (6 ounces uncooked)
¼ cup finely chopped parsley, optional

1. Heat ½ teaspoon oil in medium saucepan over medium heat until hot. Add onion and garlic. Cook and stir 2 minutes. Add tomato, peppers, ½ cup chicken broth and paprika. Reduce heat to low; cover and simmer 5 minutes.

2. Cut pork crosswise into 8 slices. Pound pork between 2 pieces of plastic wrap to ¼-inch thickness. Heat remaining ½ teaspoon oil in nonstick skillet over medium heat until hot. Cook pork 1 minute on each side or until browned. Add onion mixture. Reduce heat to low; simmer 5 minutes. Blend remaining chicken broth and flour in small bowl.

3. Remove pork from skillet; keep warm. Add flour mixture to skillet. Bring liquid to a boil; remove from heat. Stir in sour cream. Serve sauce on pork and noodles. Garnish with additional sweet Hungarian paprika and parsley, if desired. *Makes 4 servings*

NUTRIENTS PER SERVING:

Calories	380	Dietary Fiber	2 g
% calories from fat	22	Protein	28 g
Total Fat	9 g	Calcium	99 mg
Saturated Fat	2 g	Iron	5 mg
Cholesterol	110 mg	Vitamin A	412 RE
Sodium	96 mg	Vitamin C	49 mg
Carbohydrate	45 g		

Dietary Exchanges per Serving: 2½ Starch/Bread, 3 Lean Meat, 1½ Vegetable

Garlic Skewered Shrimp

2 tablespoons reduced-sodium soy sauce
1 tablespoon vegetable oil
3 cloves garlic, finely chopped
¼ teaspoon crushed red pepper (optional)
1 pound large shrimp, peeled and deveined
3 green onions, cut into 1-inch pieces

1. Soak 4 (12-inch) bamboo skewers in water 20 minutes. Combine soy sauce, oil, garlic and crushed red pepper in large resealable plastic food storage bag; add shrimp. Seal bag; turn to coat. Marinate at room temperature 10 to 15 minutes, turning occasionally.

2. Preheat broiler. Drain shrimp; reserve marinade. Alternately thread shrimp and onions onto skewers. Spray rack of broiler pan with nonstick cooking spray. Place skewers on rack. Brush with reserved marinade; discard remaining marinade. Broil 4 inches from heat, 10 minutes or until shrimp are opaque, turning occasionally. Serve on lettuce-lined plate. Garnish, if desired. *Makes 4 servings*

NUTRIENTS PER SERVING:

Calories	102	Dietary Fiber	<1 g
% calories from fat	19	Protein	19 g
Total Fat	2 g	Calcium	39 mg
Saturated Fat	<1 g	Iron	3 mg
Cholesterol	174 mg	Vitamin A	90 RE
Sodium	287 mg	Vitamin C	4 mg
Carbohydrate	<1 g		

Dietary Exchanges per Serving: 2 Lean Meat

Pork with Sweet Hungarian Paprika

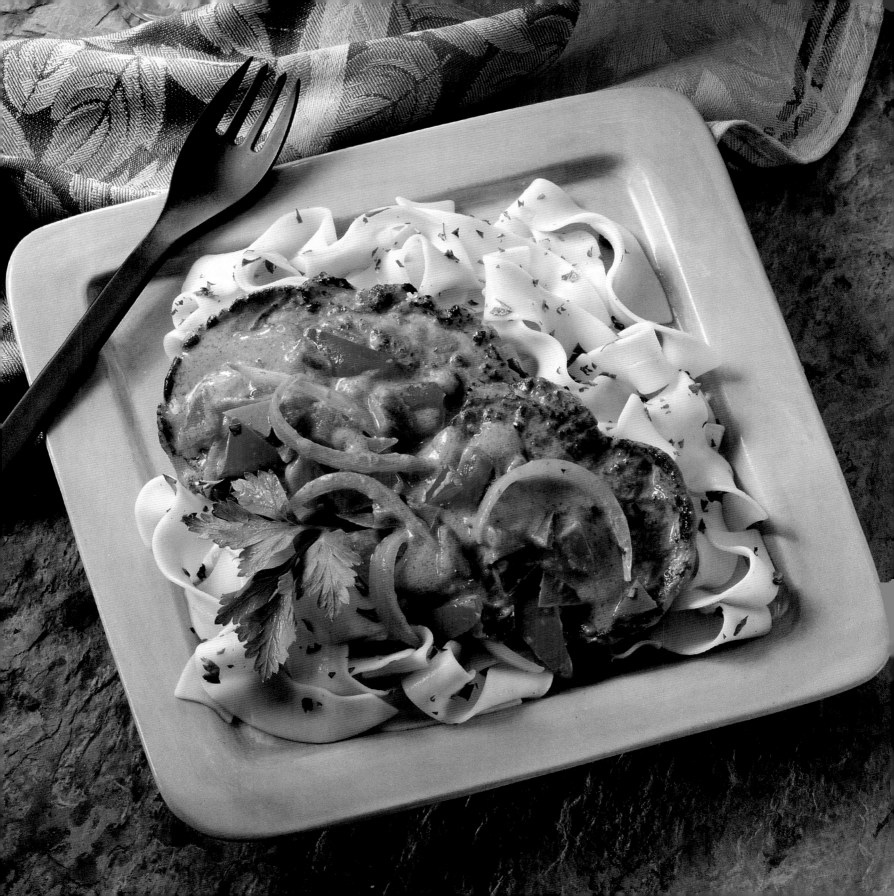

Turkey & Zucchini Enchiladas with Tomatillo and Green Chile Sauce

1 (1¼-pound) turkey leg
  Tomatillo and Green Chile Sauce (recipe follows)
1 tablespoon olive oil
1 small onion, thinly sliced
1 tablespoon finely chopped garlic
1 pound zucchini, quartered lengthwise, sliced thinly crosswise
1½ teaspoons ground cumin
½ teaspoon dried oregano leaves
¾ cup (3 ounces) shredded reduced-fat Monterey Jack cheese
12 (6-inch) corn tortillas
  Nonstick cooking spray
½ cup crumbled feta cheese

1. Place turkey in large saucepan; cover with water. Bring to a boil over high heat. Reduce heat to medium-low. Cover; simmer 1½ to 2 hours or until meat pulls apart easily when tested with fork. Drain; discard skin and bone. Cut meat into small pieces. Place in large bowl; set aside. Meanwhile, prepare Tomatillo and Green Chile Sauce.

2. Preheat oven to 350°F. Heat oil in large skillet over medium-high heat until hot. Add onion; cook and stir 3 to 4 minutes or until tender. Reduce heat to medium. Add garlic; cook and stir 5 minutes or until tender. Add zucchini, 2 tablespoons water, cumin and oregano. Cover; cook and stir over medium heat 10 minutes or until zucchini is tender. Add to turkey. Stir in Monterey Jack cheese.

3. Heat large nonstick skillet over medium-high heat until hot. Place 1 inch water in medium bowl. Dip 1 tortilla into water; shake off excess. Place in hot skillet; cook 10 to 15 seconds on each side or until tortilla is hot and pliable. Repeat with remaining tortillas.

4. Spray 13×9-inch baking pan with cooking spray. Spoon ¼ cup filling down center of each tortilla; fold sides over to enclose. Place seam side down in pan. Brush tops with ½ cup Tomatillo and Green Chile Sauce. Cover; bake 30 minutes. Top with remaining Tomatillo and Green Chile Sauce and feta cheese. Garnish with cilantro, if desired.   *Makes 6 servings*

Tomatillo and Green Chile Sauce

¾ pound fresh tomatillos *or* 2 cans (18 ounces each) whole tomatillos, drained
1 can (4 ounces) diced mild green chilies, drained
½ cup fat-free reduced-sodium chicken broth*
1 teaspoon dried oregano leaves
½ teaspoon ground cumin
2 tablespoons chopped fresh cilantro (optional)

*Omit if using canned tomatillos.

1. Place tomatillos in large saucepan; cover with water. Bring to a boil over high heat. Reduce heat to medium-high; simmer 20 to 30 minutes or until tomatillos are tender.

2. Combine tomatillos and remaining ingredients in food processor; process until smooth. Return to pan. Cover; bring to a boil over medium heat. Stir in cilantro, if desired.   *Makes about 3 cups*

NUTRIENTS PER SERVING:
includes Tomatillo and Green Chile Sauce

Calories	377	Dietary Fiber	5 g
% calories from fat	28	Protein	29 g
Total Fat	12 g	Calcium	320 mg
Saturated Fat	3 g	Iron	4 mg
Cholesterol	48 mg	Vitamin A	76 RE
Sodium	284 mg	Vitamin C	34 mg
Carbohydrate	41 g		

Dietary Exchanges per Serving: 1½ Starch/Bread, 1½ Lean Meat, 1 Fruit

Beef & Vegetable Stir-Fry

½ cup fat-free reduced-sodium beef broth
3 tablespoons reduced-sodium soy sauce
2 teaspoons cornstarch
1 teaspoon sugar
½ teaspoon ground ginger
½ teaspoon garlic powder
½ teaspoon Oriental sesame oil
¼ teaspoon salt
¼ teaspoon ground black pepper
1 teaspoon vegetable oil
½ pound beef flank steak, cut diagonally into
  1-inch slices
2 green bell peppers, thinly sliced
1 tomato, cut into wedges
8 green onions, cut into 1-inch pieces
4 cups hot cooked white rice (optional)

1. Blend beef broth, soy sauce, cornstarch, sugar, ginger, garlic powder, sesame oil, salt and black pepper in medium bowl.

2. Heat vegetable oil in wok or large nonstick skillet over medium-high heat until hot. Add beef; stir-fry 3 minutes or until beef is browned. Add bell peppers, tomato and onions; stir-fry 2 minutes or until vegetables are crisp-tender.

3. Stir beef broth mixture; add to wok. Cook and stir 3 minutes or until sauce boils and thickens.

4. Serve beef mixture over hot cooked white rice, if desired. *Makes 4 servings*

NUTRIENTS PER SERVING:

Calories	357	Dietary Fiber	2 g
% calories from fat	15	Protein	19 g
Total Fat	6 g	Calcium	35 mg
Saturated Fat	2 g	Iron	4 mg
Cholesterol	23 mg	Vitamin A	108 RE
Sodium	614 mg	Vitamin C	48 mg
Carbohydrate	54 g		

Dietary Exchanges per Serving: 2½ Starch/Bread, 2 Lean Meat, 2 Vegetable

Turkey Jambalaya

1 teaspoon vegetable oil
1 cup chopped onion
1 green bell pepper, chopped
½ cup chopped celery
3 cloves garlic, finely chopped
1¾ cups fat-free reduced-sodium chicken broth
1 cup chopped seeded tomato
¼ pound ground turkey breast, cooked
¼ pound turkey sausage, cooked
3 tablespoons tomato paste
1 bay leaf
1 teaspoon dried basil leaves
¼ teaspoon ground red pepper
1 cup uncooked white rice
¼ cup chopped fresh parsley

1. Heat oil in large nonstick skillet over medium-high heat until hot. Add onion, bell pepper, celery and garlic. Cook and stir 5 minutes or until vegetables are tender.

2. Add chicken broth, tomato, turkey, turkey sausage, tomato paste, bay leaf, basil and red pepper. Stir in rice. Bring to a boil over high heat, stirring occasionally. Cover, reduce heat to medium-low. Simmer 20 minutes or until rice is tender.

3. Remove skillet from heat. Remove and discard bay leaf. Top servings evenly with parsley. Serve immediately. *Makes 4 servings*

NUTRIENTS PER SERVING:

Calories	416	Dietary Fiber	3 g
% calories from fat	18	Protein	28 g
Total Fat	9 g	Calcium	84 mg
Saturated Fat	2 g	Iron	5 mg
Cholesterol	74 mg	Vitamin A	306 RE
Sodium	384 mg	Vitamin C	44 mg
Carbohydrate	51 g		

Dietary Exchanges per Serving: 2½ Starch/Bread, 2 Lean Meat, 2½ Vegetable, ½ Fat

Chicken Breasts with Crabmeat Stuffing

4 boneless skinless chicken breast halves (about 1 pound)
3 ounces canned crabmeat, rinsed and drained
¾ cup whole wheat cracker crumbs, divided
¼ cup fat-free mayonnaise
2 tablespoons grated Parmesan cheese
2 tablespoons finely chopped green onion
2 tablespoons fresh lemon juice
¼ teaspoon hot pepper sauce
1 tablespoon dried parsley flakes
1 teaspoon coarsely ground black pepper
1 teaspoon paprika
½ cup 1% low-fat milk

1. **Microwave Directions:** Pound chicken breasts to ¼-inch thickness.

2. Combine crabmeat, ¼ cup cracker crumbs, mayonnaise, cheese, onion, lemon juice and pepper sauce in medium bowl. Spoon filling onto chicken breasts. Roll up each chicken breast from short side, tucking in ends; secure with wooden pick.

3. Combine remaining ½ cup cracker crumbs, parsley, pepper and paprika. Dip chicken in milk; roll in cracker crumb mixture. Place chicken in microwavable round or square baking dish. Cover with waxed paper. Microwave at HIGH 10 minutes or until chicken is no longer pink in center. Remove chicken from dish. Add remaining milk to pan juices; microwave at HIGH 1 minute or until sauce comes to a boil. Serve chicken with sauce.   *Makes 4 servings*

NUTRIENTS PER SERVING:

Calories	246	Dietary Fiber	<1 g
% calories from fat	17	Protein	30 g
Total Fat	5 g	Calcium	113 mg
Saturated Fat	2 g	Iron	2 mg
Cholesterol	83 mg	Vitamin A	67 RE
Sodium	424 mg	Vitamin C	6 mg
Carbohydrate	21 g		

Dietary Exchanges per Serving: 1½ Starch/Bread, 3 Lean Meat

Paella

10 ounces boneless skinless chicken breasts
1 teaspoon vegetable oil
½ cup uncooked white rice
4 cloves garlic, finely chopped
½ cup sliced onion
½ cup sliced green bell pepper
1 cup fat-free reduced-sodium chicken broth
½ teaspoon ground turmeric
¼ teaspoon salt
¼ teaspoon paprika
¼ teaspoon ground black pepper
½ cup frozen green peas
½ cup drained canned diced tomatoes
8 ounces medium shrimp, peeled

1. Preheat oven to 350°F. Spray large nonstick skillet with nonstick cooking spray. Add chicken. Cook 10 minutes or until chicken is no longer pink in center, turning once. Remove chicken from skillet. Cool 10 minutes or until cool enough to handle. Cut into 1-inch pieces.

2. Heat oil in large ovenproof skillet or paella pan over medium heat until hot. Add rice and garlic. Cook 5 minutes or until rice is lightly browned, stirring occasionally. Add onion and bell pepper. Stir in chicken broth, turmeric, salt, paprika and black pepper. Stir in peas and tomatoes. Place chicken and shrimp on top of rice mixture.

3. Bake 20 minutes or until heated through. Let stand 5 minutes before serving.   *Makes 4 servings*

NUTRIENTS PER SERVING:

Calories	258	Dietary Fiber	2 g
% calories from fat	14	Protein	27 g
Total Fat	4 g	Calcium	51 mg
Saturated Fat	1 g	Iron	4 mg
Cholesterol	123 mg	Vitamin A	95 RE
Sodium	371 mg	Vitamin C	36 mg
Carbohydrate	28 g		

Dietary Exchanges per Serving: 1½ Starch/Bread, 3 Lean Meat, 1 Vegetable

Chicken Breasts with Crabmeat Stuffing

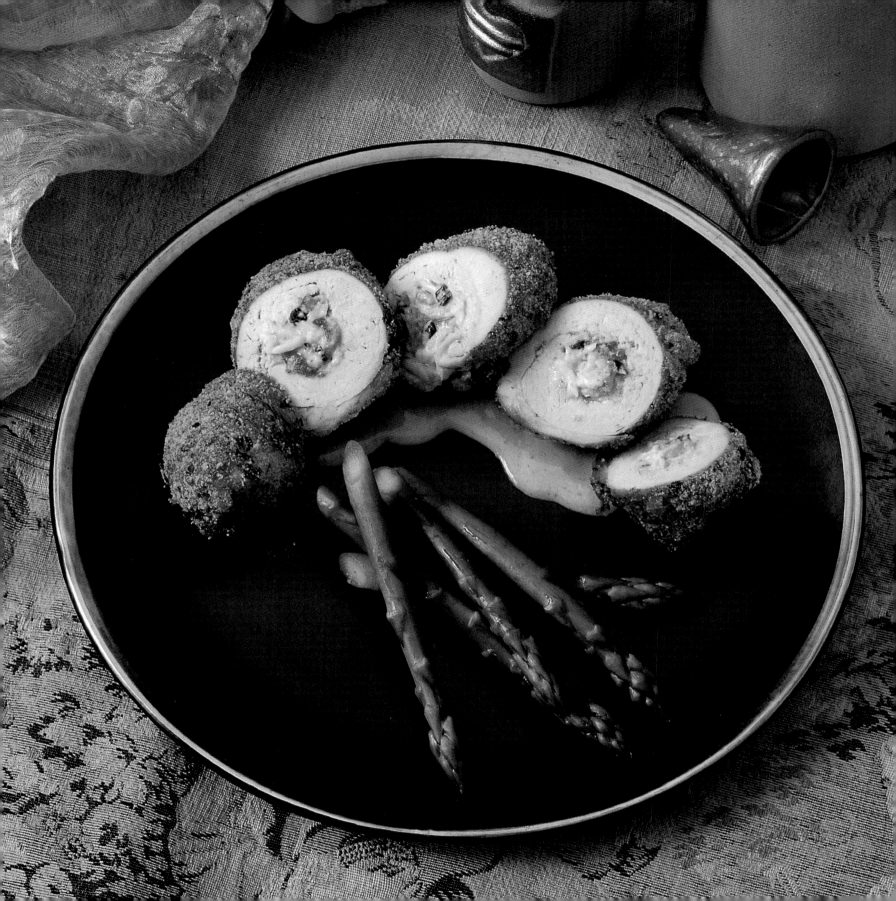

Stir-Fried Pork Lo Mein

Nonstick cooking spray
6 green onions, cut into 1-inch pieces
½ teaspoon garlic powder
½ teaspoon ground ginger
6 ounces pork loin roast, thinly sliced
3 cups shredded green cabbage
½ cup shredded carrots
½ cup trimmed snow peas
½ cup fat-free reduced-sodium chicken broth
2 teaspoons cornstarch
2 tablespoons hoisin sauce (optional)
1 tablespoon reduced-sodium soy sauce
8 ounces hot cooked linguine

1. Spray wok or large nonstick skillet with cooking spray. Heat over medium heat until hot. Add onions, garlic powder and ginger; stir-fry 30 seconds. Add pork; stir-fry 2 minutes or until pork is no longer pink. Add vegetables; stir-fry 3 minutes or until vegetables are crisp-tender.

2. Blend chicken broth, cornstarch, hoisin sauce, if desired, and soy sauce in small bowl. Add to wok. Cook and stir until mixture boils and thickens. Serve vegetables and sauce over pasta.   *Makes 4 servings*

NUTRIENTS PER SERVING:

Calories	310	Dietary Fiber	4 g
% calories from fat	13	Protein	20 g
Total Fat	4 g	Calcium	66 mg
Saturated Fat	1 g	Iron	3 mg
Cholesterol	25 mg	Vitamin A	445 RE
Sodium	228 mg	Vitamin C	48 mg
Carbohydrate	48 g		

Dietary Exchanges per Serving: 3 Starch/Bread, 1 Lean Meat, 1½ Vegetable

Bow Tie Pasta with Puttanesca Sauce

1 teaspoon olive oil
3 cloves garlic, finely chopped
1 can (28 ounces) crushed Italian-style tomatoes, undrained
1 can (9 ounces) water-packed white tuna, rinsed and drained
¼ cup sliced black olives
¼ teaspoon crushed red pepper
¼ teaspoon ground black pepper
8 ounces hot, cooked bow tie pasta

1. Heat oil in large saucepan over medium-high heat until hot. Add garlic. Cook and stir 3 minutes. Stir in remaining ingredients except pasta. Reduce heat to medium-low. Simmer 5 minutes, stirring occasionally.

2. Serve sauce on pasta. Serve immediately.

Makes 4 servings

NUTRIENTS PER SERVING:

Calories	351	Dietary Fiber	4 g
% calories from fat	17	Protein	26 g
Total Fat	7 g	Calcium	80 mg
Saturated Fat	1 g	Iron	4 mg
Cholesterol	19 mg	Vitamin A	143 RE
Sodium	825 mg	Vitamin C	31 mg
Carbohydrate	47 g		

Dietary Exchanges per Serving: 2½ Starch/Bread, 2 Lean Meat, 2 Vegetable

Stir-Fried Pork Lo Mein

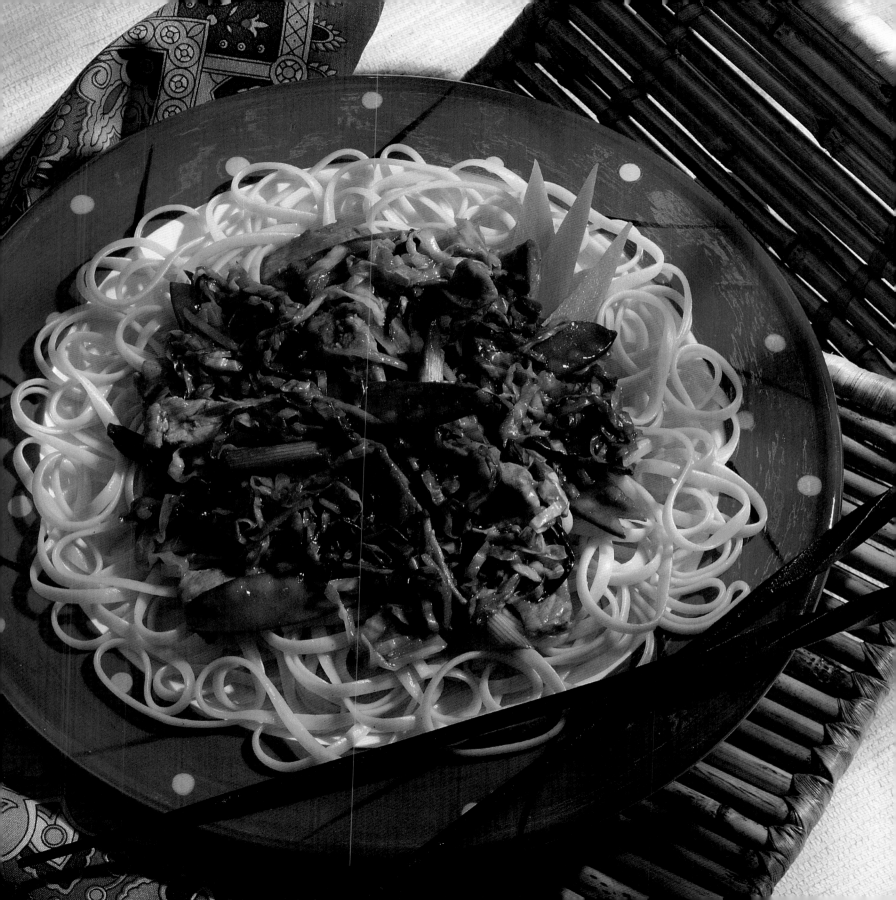

Pad Thai

8 ounces uncooked rice noodles, ⅛ inch wide
1½ tablespoons fish sauce*
1 to 2 tablespoons fresh lemon juice
2 tablespoons rice wine vinegar
1 tablespoon ketchup
2 teaspoons sugar
¼ teaspoon crushed red pepper
1 tablespoon vegetable oil
4 ounces boneless skinless chicken breast, finely chopped
2 green onions, thinly sliced
2 cloves garlic, finely chopped
3 ounces small shrimp, peeled
2 cups fresh bean sprouts
1 medium carrot, shredded
3 tablespoons finely chopped fresh cilantro
2 tablespoons chopped unsalted dry-roasted peanuts

*Fish sauce is available at most larger supermarkets and Oriental markets.

1. Place noodles in medium bowl. Cover with lukewarm water; let stand 30 minutes or until soft. Drain; set aside. Whisk fish sauce, lemon juice, vinegar, ketchup, sugar and pepper in small bowl; set aside.

2. Heat oil in wok or large nonstick skillet over medium-high heat. Add chicken, green onions and garlic. Cook and stir until chicken is no longer pink. Stir in noodles; cook 1 minute. Add shrimp and bean sprouts; cook just until shrimp turn opaque, about 3 minutes. Stir in fish sauce mixture; toss to coat. Cook until heated through, about 2 minutes.

3. Arrange noodle mixture on platter; sprinkle with carrot, cilantro and peanuts. Garnish with lemon wedges, tomato wedges and fresh cilantro, if desired.

Makes 5 servings

NUTRIENTS PER SERVING:

Calories	265	Dietary Fiber	1 g
% calories from fat	18	Protein	14 g
Total Fat	6 g	Calcium	78 mg
Saturated Fat	1 g	Iron	2 mg
Cholesterol	38 mg	Vitamin A	453 RE
Sodium	798 mg	Vitamin C	13 mg
Carbohydrate	42 g		

Dietary Exchanges per Serving: 2½ Starch/Bread, ½ Lean Meat, 1 Vegetable, ½ Fat

Cook's Tip: To peel garlic easily, place a clove on a cutting board. Cover the clove with the flat side of a chef's knife blade, then firmly press down on the blade with your fist. This loosens the skin so that it comes right off.

Pad Thai

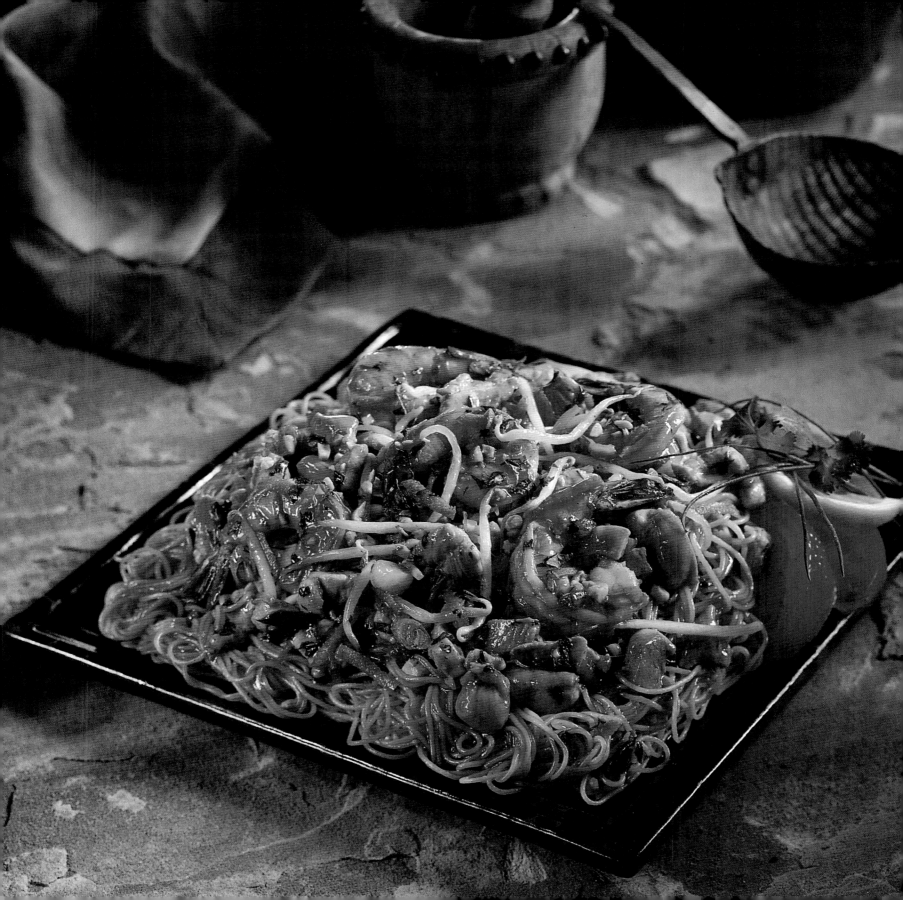

Cheese Ravioli with Pumpkin Sauce

Nonstick cooking spray
⅓ cup sliced green onions
1 to 2 cloves garlic, finely chopped
½ teaspoon fennel seeds
1 cup evaporated skim milk
1 tablespoon all-purpose flour
¼ teaspoon salt
⅛ teaspoon ground black pepper
½ cup solid pack pumpkin
2 packages (9 ounces each) refrigerated low-fat cheese ravioli
2 tablespoons grated Parmesan cheese (optional)

1. Generously spray medium nonstick saucepan with cooking spray; heat over medium heat until hot. Add onions, garlic and fennel seeds; cook and stir 3 minutes or until onions are tender.

2. Blend milk, flour, salt and pepper in small bowl until smooth; stir into saucepan. Bring to a boil over high heat; boil until thickened, stirring constantly. Stir in pumpkin; reduce heat to low.

3. Meanwhile, cook pasta according to package directions, omitting salt. Drain. Divide ravioli evenly among 6 plates. Top with pumpkin sauce and sprinkle with cheese, if desired. Serve immediately. Garnish as desired. *Makes 6 servings*

NUTRIENTS PER SERVING:

Calories	270	Dietary Fiber	1 g
% calories from fat	7	Protein	18 g
Total Fat	2 g	Calcium	135 mg
Saturated Fat	1 g	Iron	1 mg
Cholesterol	6 mg	Vitamin A	522 RE
Sodium	556 mg	Vitamin C	4 mg
Carbohydrate	45 g		

Dietary Exchanges per Serving: 2½ Starch/Bread, 1 Lean Meat, ½ Milk

Beef Burritos

Nonstick cooking spray
10 ounces lean ground beef
½ cup chopped onion
3 cloves garlic, finely chopped
1 can (14½ ounces) Mexican-style diced tomatoes, drained
1 package (10 ounces) frozen whole kernel corn
¼ cup drained canned diced mild green chilies
1 tablespoon chili powder
1 teaspoon ground cumin
4 (6-inch) flour tortillas

1. Spray large nonstick skillet with cooking spray. Heat over medium-high heat until hot. Add beef, onion and garlic. Cook and stir 5 minutes or until beef is no longer pink. Add tomatoes, corn, chilies, chili powder and cumin. Cook 5 minutes or until heated through, stirring occasionally.

2. Spoon beef mixture evenly down center of each tortilla. Fold bottoms of tortillas over fillings. Roll up burritos. Serve immediately. *Makes 4 servings*

NUTRIENTS PER SERVING:

Calories	338	Dietary Fiber	4 g
% calories from fat	28	Protein	20 g
Total Fat	11 g	Calcium	51 mg
Saturated Fat	4 g	Iron	3 mg
Cholesterol	44 mg	Vitamin A	153 RE
Sodium	333 mg	Vitamin C	26 mg
Carbohydrate	43 g		

Dietary Exchanges per Serving: 2 Starch/Bread, 2 Lean Meat, 2½ Vegetable, ½ Fat

Cheese Ravioli with Pumpkin Sauce

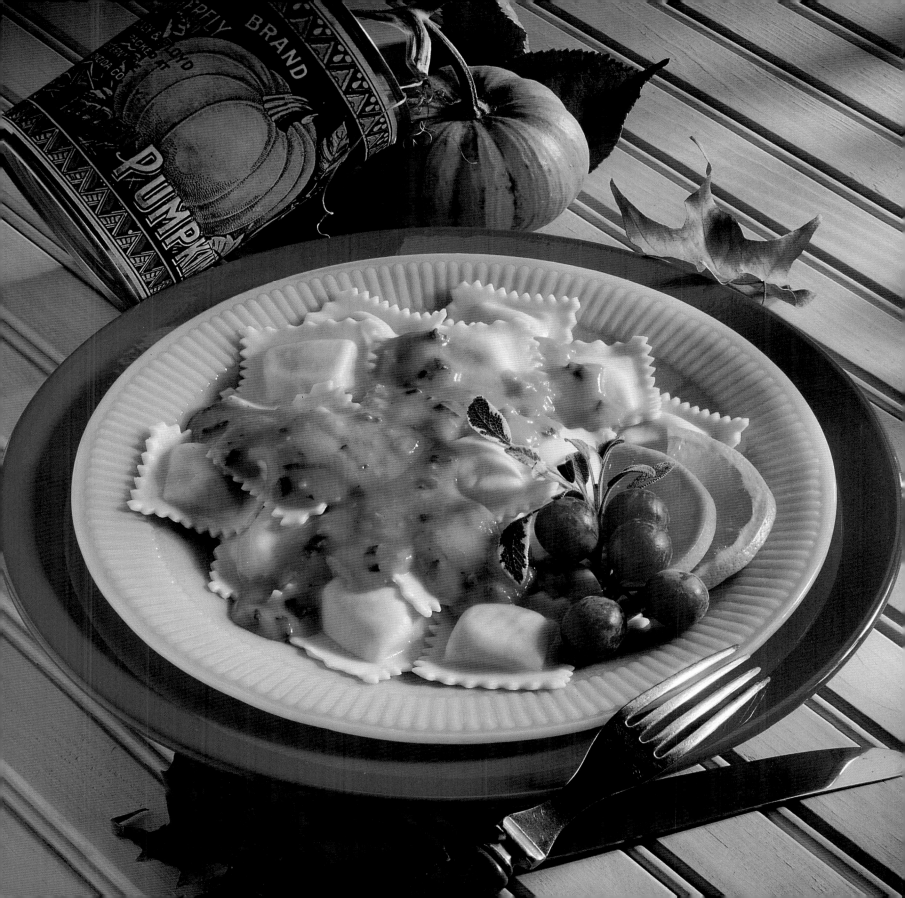

Greek White Bean Risotto

**3 teaspoons low-sodium chicken flavor bouillon
granules**
Nonstick cooking spray
3 cloves garlic, finely chopped
1½ cups uncooked arborio rice
2 teaspoons dried oregano leaves
**⅓ cup finely chopped solid-pack sun-dried
tomatoes**
**1 cup rinsed, drained canned white kidney
beans**
¾ cup (3 ounces) crumbled feta cheese
⅓ cup shredded Parmesan cheese
1 teaspoon lemon juice
½ teaspoon ground black pepper

1. Combine 5½ cups water and bouillon granules in large saucepan; cover. Bring to a simmer over medium-low heat.

2. Spray another large saucepan with cooking spray; heat over medium heat until hot. Add garlic; cook and stir 1 minute. Add rice and oregano; reduce heat to medium-low.

3. Add 1 cup hot broth to saucepan; cook until broth is absorbed, stirring constantly. Add ½ cup hot broth to rice mixture, stirring constantly until broth is absorbed. Stir tomatoes into rice mixture. Stir remaining hot broth into rice mixture, ½ cup at a time, stirring constantly until all broth is absorbed before adding next ½ cup. (Total cooking time is about 35 to 40 minutes or until rice is just tender but still firm to the bite.)

4. Add beans; cook 1 minute, stirring constantly. Remove from heat. Stir in cheeses, lemon juice and pepper. Cover; let stand 5 minutes. Stir once. Serve with breadsticks and garnish, if desired.

Makes 5 servings

NUTRIENTS PER SERVING:

Calories	351	Dietary Fiber	3 g
% calories from fat	17	Protein	13 g
Total Fat	7 g	Calcium	211 mg
Saturated Fat	4 g	Iron	4 mg
Cholesterol	20 mg	Vitamin A	235 RE
Sodium	831 mg	Vitamin C	6 mg
Carbohydrate	60 g		

Dietary Exchanges per Serving: 4 Starch/Bread,
1 Lean Meat, ½ Fat

Health Note: An estimated 50 percent of older adults rely on nonbulk forming laxatives for regularity. Frequent use of these laxatives lowers the level of the blood protein albumin. Research suggests that lower than normal albumin levels may increase your risk of heart disease and cancer. Instead, try a more natural approach to regularity—increase your intake of fluids and fiber-rich foods, such as beans, whole grains, fruits and vegetables, and increase your level of physical activity.

Greek White Bean Risotto

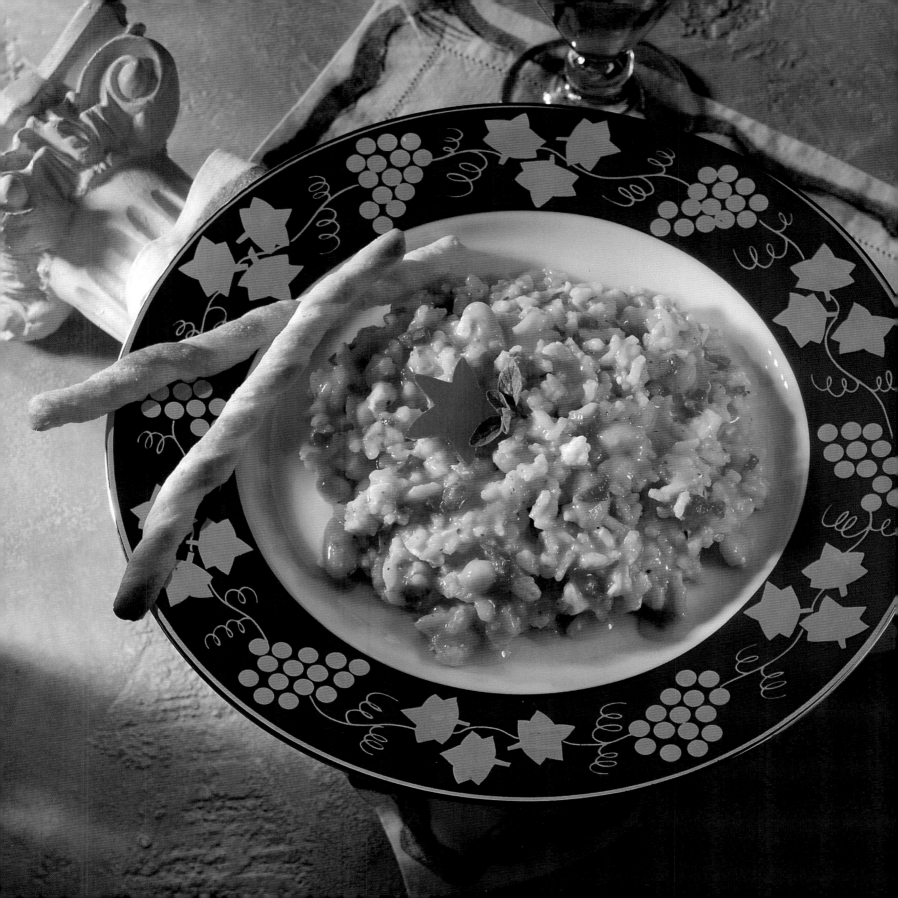

Shrimp & Snow Peas with Fusilli

6 ounces uncooked fusilli
Nonstick cooking spray
2 cloves garlic, finely chopped
¼ teaspoon crushed red pepper
12 ounces medium shrimp, peeled
2 cups snow peas
1 can (8 ounces) sliced water chestnuts, drained
⅓ cup sliced green onions
3 tablespoons lime juice
2 tablespoons chopped fresh cilantro
2 tablespoons olive oil
1 tablespoon reduced-sodium soy sauce
1½ teaspoons Mexican seasoning

1. Cook pasta according to package directions, omitting salt; drain. Set aside.

2. Spray large nonstick skillet with cooking spray; heat over medium heat until hot. Add garlic and red pepper; stir-fry 1 minute. Add shrimp; stir-fry 5 minutes or until shrimp are opaque. Remove shrimp from skillet.

3. Add snow peas and 2 tablespoons water to skillet; cook, covered, 1 minute. Uncover; cook and stir 2 minutes or until snow peas are crisp-tender. Remove snow peas from skillet.

4. Combine pasta, shrimp, snow peas, water chestnuts and onions in large bowl. Blend lime juice, cilantro, oil, soy sauce and Mexican seasoning in small bowl. Drizzle over pasta mixture; toss to coat. Garnish with radishes, if desired. *Makes 6 servings*

NUTRIENTS PER SERVING:

Calories	228	Dietary Fiber	3 g
% calories from fat	24	Protein	15 g
Total Fat	6 g	Calcium	52 mg
Saturated Fat	1 g	Iron	4 mg
Cholesterol	87 mg	Vitamin A	92 RE
Sodium	202 mg	Vitamin C	36 mg
Carbohydrate	29 g		

Dietary Exchanges per Serving: 1½ Starch/Bread, 1 Lean Meat, 1 Vegetable, 1 Fat

Health Note: Recent studies have shown that garlic may play a role in the prevention of heart disease. Results indicate that a clove of garlic a day may lower levels of bad cholesterol (LDL), may help prevent the formation of blood clots that lead to heart attacks and strokes, and may aid in lowering high blood pressure levels.

Shrimp & Snow Peas with Fusilli

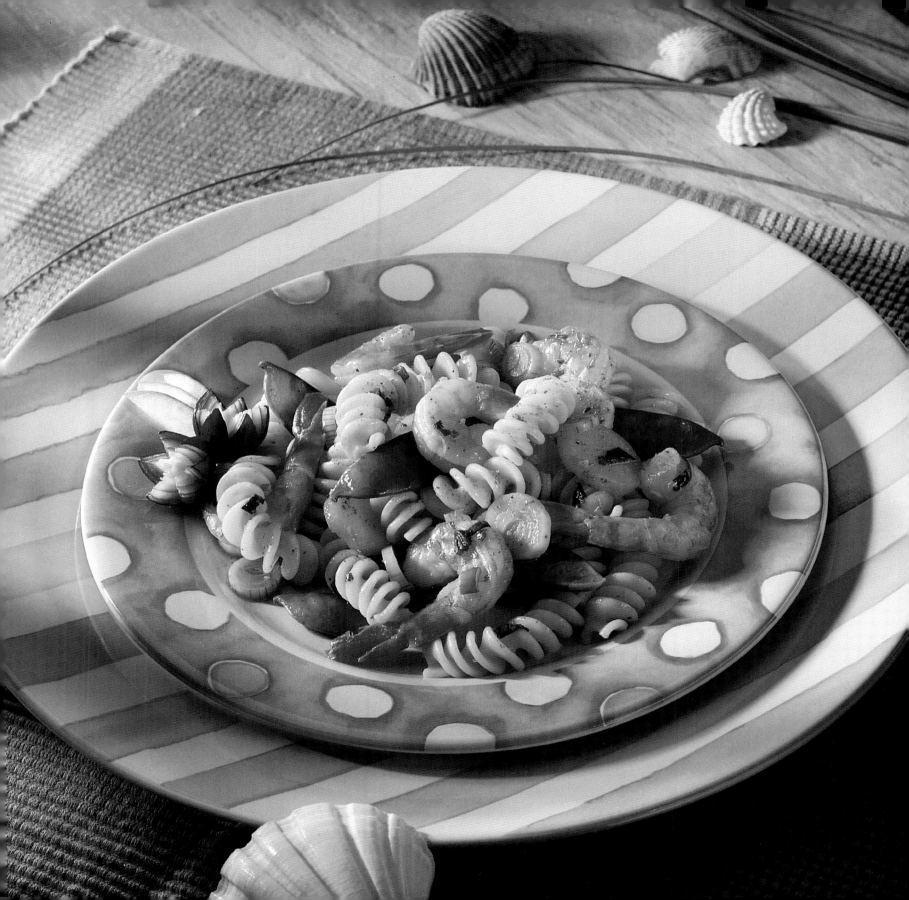

Chicken Fajitas with Cowpoke Barbecue Sauce

1 cup Cowpoke Barbecue Sauce (recipe follows), divided
10 ounces boneless skinless chicken breasts, cut lengthwise into 1×½-inch pieces
2 green or red bell peppers, thinly sliced
1 cup sliced onion
2 cups tomato wedges
4 (6-inch) flour tortillas, warmed

1. Prepare Cowpoke Barbecue Sauce. Spray large nonstick skillet with nonstick cooking spray. Heat over medium-high heat until hot. Brush chicken with ¼ cup barbecue sauce. Add to skillet. Cook and stir 3 minutes or until chicken is browned. Add peppers and onion. Cook and stir 3 minutes or until vegetables are crisp-tender and chicken is no longer pink. Add tomatoes. Cook 2 minutes or until heated through, stirring occasionally.

2. Serve with warm flour tortillas and remaining ¾ cup Cowpoke Barbecue Sauce. Garnish with cilantro, if desired.   *Makes 4 servings*

NUTRIENTS PER SERVING:

Calories	310	Dietary Fiber	4 g
% calories from fat	18	Protein	20 g
Total Fat	6 g	Calcium	104 mg
Saturated Fat	1 g	Iron	3 mg
Cholesterol	36 mg	Vitamin A	259 RE
Sodium	736 mg	Vitamin C	90 mg
Carbohydrate	47 g		

Dietary Exchanges per Serving: 1½ Starch/Bread, 2 Lean Meat, 2½ Vegetable

Cowpoke Barbecue Sauce

1 teaspoon vegetable oil
¾ cup chopped green onions
3 cloves garlic, finely chopped
1 can (14½ ounces) crushed tomatoes
½ cup ketchup
¼ cup water
¼ cup orange juice
2 tablespoons cider vinegar
2 teaspoons chili sauce
Dash Worcestershire sauce

Heat oil in large nonstick saucepan over medium heat until hot. Add onions and garlic. Cook and stir 5 minutes or until onions are tender. Stir in remaining ingredients. Reduce heat to medium-low. Cook 15 minutes, stirring occasionally.   *Makes 2 cups*

Chicken Fajitas with Cowpoke Barbecue Sauce

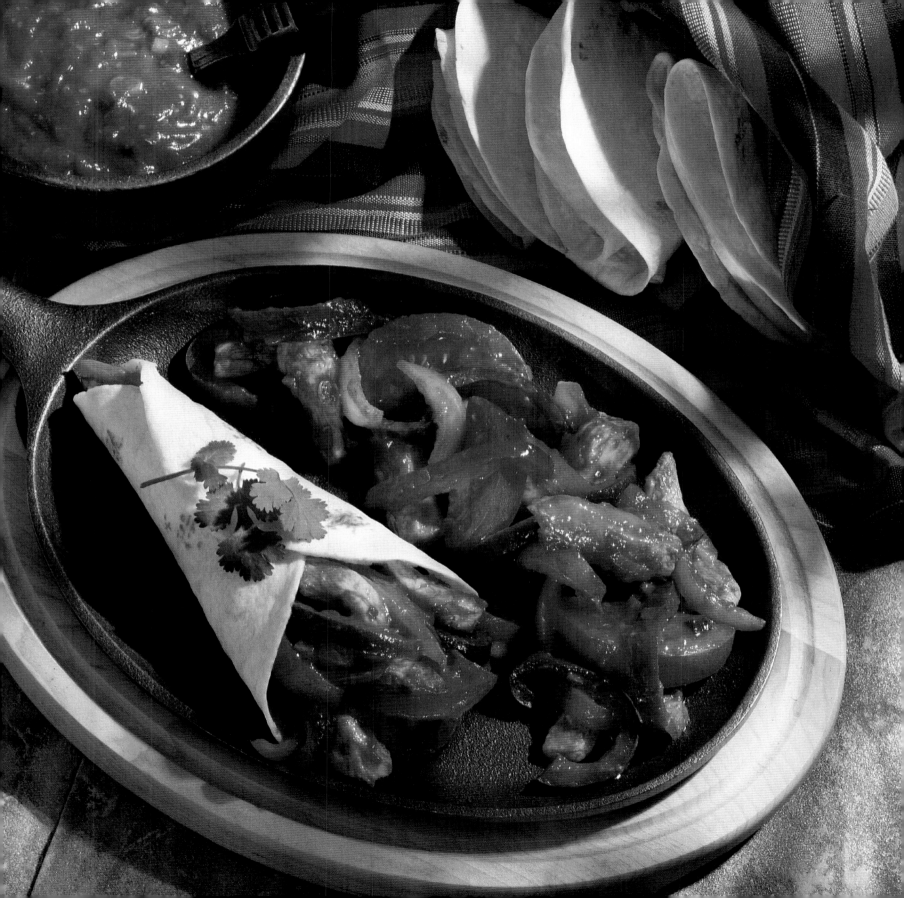

Tamale Pie

BISCUIT TOPPING
  ½ **cup white or yellow cornmeal**
  ½ **cup buttermilk**
  ⅓ **cup all-purpose flour**
  1 **egg white, slightly beaten**
  1 **tablespoon sugar**
  ½ **jalapeño pepper, seeded, chopped***
  1 **teaspoon baking powder**

FILLING
  Nonstick cooking spray
  1 **green bell pepper, chopped**
  ¾ **cup chopped green onions**
  2 **cloves garlic, finely chopped**
 1½ **cups canned crushed tomatoes**
  1 **can (about 15 ounces) pinto beans, rinsed**
     and drained
  ¼ **pound cooked ground turkey breast**
  2 **teaspoons chili powder**
  1 **teaspoon ground cumin**
  ¼ **teaspoon ground black pepper**

*Jalapeño peppers can sting and irritate the skin. Wear rubber gloves when handling peppers and do not touch eyes.

1. Preheat oven to 425°F. Spray 9-inch pie plate with nonstick cooking spray; set aside.

2. For topping, combine all topping ingredients in large bowl until well blended; set aside.

3. For filling, spray large nonstick skillet with cooking spray. Heat over medium heat until hot. Add bell pepper, onions and garlic. Cook and stir 5 minutes or until vegetables are tender. Add tomatoes, beans, turkey, chili powder, cumin and black pepper. Cook and stir 5 minutes or until heated through.

4. Spoon vegetable mixture into prepared pie plate. Drop heaping tablespoonfuls topping around outer edge of filling; flatten with back of spoon to form biscuits.

5. Bake 25 minutes or until biscuits are golden brown. Let stand 5 minutes before serving.   *Makes 4 servings*

NUTRIENTS PER SERVING:

Calories	274	Dietary Fiber	4 g
% calories from fat	13	Protein	14 g
Total Fat	4 g	Calcium	140 mg
Saturated Fat	1 g	Iron	5 mg
Cholesterol	12 mg	Vitamin A	199 RE
Sodium	750 mg	Vitamin C	45 mg
Carbohydrate	47 g		

Dietary Exchanges per Serving: 2½ Starch/Bread, 1 Lean Meat, 1 Vegetable

Grilled Tuna Niçoise with Citrus Marinade

  Citrus Marinade (page 79)
  1 **tuna steak (about 1 pound)**
  2 **cups green beans, trimmed, halved**
  4 **cups romaine lettuce leaves, washed, torn**
     into small pieces
  8 **small red potatoes, cooked and quartered**
  1 **cup chopped seeded tomato**
  4 **hard-cooked egg whites, chopped**
  ¼ **cup sliced red onion, halved**
  2 **teaspoons chopped black olives**
  Low-calorie salad dressing (optional)

1. Prepare Citrus Marinade; combine with tuna in large resealable plastic food storage bag. Seal bag; turn to coat. Marinate in refrigerator 1 hour, turning occasionally.* Drain tuna; discard marinade.

2. To prevent sticking, spray grill with nonstick cooking spray. Prepare coals for grilling.

*Marinate in refrigerator 1 hour for each inch of thickness.

3. Place tuna on grill, 4 inches from hot coals. Grill 8 to 10 minutes or until tuna flakes easily when tested with fork, turning once. Or, place tuna on rack of broiler pan coated with nonstick cooking spray. Broil 4 inches from heat, 8 to 10 minutes or until tuna flakes easily when tested with fork. Slice tuna into ¼-inch-thick slices; set aside.

4. Place 2 cups water in large saucepan; bring to a boil over high heat. Add beans; cook 2 minutes. Drain; rinse with cold water and drain again.

5. Place lettuce on large serving platter. Arrange tuna, beans, potatoes, tomato, egg whites and onion on lettuce. Sprinkle with olives. Serve with low calorie salad dressing, if desired. *Makes 4 servings*

Citrus Marinade

½ cup fresh lime juice
¼ cup vegetable oil
2 green onions, chopped
1 teaspoon dried tarragon leaves
¼ teaspoon garlic powder
¼ teaspoon ground black pepper

Blend all ingredients in small bowl.

NUTRIENTS PER SERVING:

Calories	373	Dietary Fiber	6 g
% calories from fat	16	Protein	35 g
Total Fat	7 g	Calcium	92 mg
Saturated Fat	1 g	Iron	4 mg
Cholesterol	48 mg	Vitamin A	246 RE
Sodium	160 mg	Vitamin C	55 mg
Carbohydrate	45 g		

Dietary Exchanges per Serving: 2 Starch/Bread,
3 Lean Meat, 2½ Vegetable

Fettuccine Alfredo

2 teaspoons margarine
3 cloves garlic, finely chopped
4½ teaspoons all-purpose flour
1½ cups skim milk
½ cup grated Parmesan cheese
3½ teaspoons Neufchâtel cheese
¼ teaspoon white pepper
4 ounces hot cooked fettuccine
¼ cup chopped fresh parsley

1. Melt margarine in medium saucepan over medium heat. Add garlic. Cook and stir 1 minute. Stir in flour. Cook and stir 2 minutes or until small clumps form. Gradually stir in milk. Cook 6 minutes or until sauce thickens, stirring constantly. Add cheeses and pepper; cook until melted, stirring constantly.

2. Serve sauce over fettuccine; top with parsley. Garnish as desired. *Makes 4 servings*

NUTRIENTS PER SERVING:

Calories	242	Dietary Fiber	1 g
% calories from fat	33	Protein	14 g
Total Fat	9 g	Calcium	307 mg
Saturated Fat	4 g	Iron	1 mg
Cholesterol	18 mg	Vitamin A	160 RE
Sodium	344 mg	Vitamin C	7 mg
Carbohydrate	27 g		

Dietary Exchanges per Serving: 2 Starch/Bread,
1 Lean Meat, 1 Fat

Cashew Chicken

10 ounces boneless skinless chicken breasts, cut into 1×½-inch pieces
1 tablespoon cornstarch
1 tablespoon dry white wine
1 tablespoon reduced-sodium soy sauce
½ teaspoon garlic powder
1 teaspoon vegetable oil
6 green onions, cut into 1-inch pieces
2 cups sliced mushrooms
1 red or green bell pepper, thinly sliced
1 can (6 ounces) sliced water chestnuts, drained
2 tablespoons hoisin sauce (optional)
2 cups hot cooked white rice
¼ cup roasted cashews

1. Place chicken in large resealable plastic food storage bag. Blend cornstarch, wine, soy sauce and garlic powder in small bowl. Pour over chicken pieces. Seal bag; turn to coat. Marinate in refrigerator 1 hour. Drain chicken; discard marinade.

2. Heat oil in wok or large nonstick skillet over medium-high heat until hot. Add onions; stir-fry 1 minute. Add chicken; stir-fry 2 minutes or until browned. Add mushrooms, pepper and water chestnuts; stir-fry 3 minutes or until vegetables are crisp-tender and chicken is no longer pink in center. Stir in hoisin sauce, if desired. Cook and stir 1 minute or until heated through.

3. Serve chicken and vegetables on rice. Top servings evenly with cashews. Serve immediately.

Makes 4 servings

NUTRIENTS PER SERVING:

Calories	274	Dietary Fiber	3 g
% calories from fat	23	Protein	18 g
Total Fat	7 g	Calcium	28 mg
Saturated Fat	1 g	Iron	3 mg
Cholesterol	36 mg	Vitamin A	52 RE
Sodium	83 mg	Vitamin C	22 mg
Carbohydrate	34 g		

Dietary Exchanges per Serving: 1½ Starch/Bread, 2 Lean Meat, 1½ Vegetable, ½ Fat

Spinach-Stuffed Shells

1 package (10 ounces) chopped frozen spinach, thawed and drained
1½ cups nonfat ricotta cheese
½ cup grated Parmesan cheese
½ cup cholesterol-free egg substitute
3 cloves garlic, finely chopped
1 teaspoon dried oregano leaves
½ teaspoon salt
½ teaspoon dried basil leaves
½ teaspoon dried marjoram leaves
¼ teaspoon ground black pepper
24 large pasta shells, cooked
2 cans (14½ ounces each) crushed tomatoes
1 cup (4 ounces) shredded reduced-fat mozzarella cheese

1. Preheat oven to 350°F. Spray 13×9-inch baking pan with nonstick cooking spray.

2. Combine spinach, ricotta and Parmesan cheeses, egg substitute, garlic, oregano, salt, basil, marjoram and pepper in large bowl. Spoon into shells. Place shells in prepared pan. Top with undrained tomatoes and mozzarella cheese. Bake 20 minutes or until cheese melts.

Makes 4 servings

NUTRIENTS PER SERVING:

Calories	456	Dietary Fiber	6 g
% calories from fat	20	Protein	38 g
Total Fat	11 g	Calcium	684 mg
Saturated Fat	6 g	Iron	5 mg
Cholesterol	35 mg	Vitamin A	1,081 RE
Sodium	803 mg	Vitamin C	41 mg
Carbohydrate	57 g		

Dietary Exchanges per Serving: 3 Starch/Bread, 3 Lean Meat, 2 Vegetable

Cashew Chicken

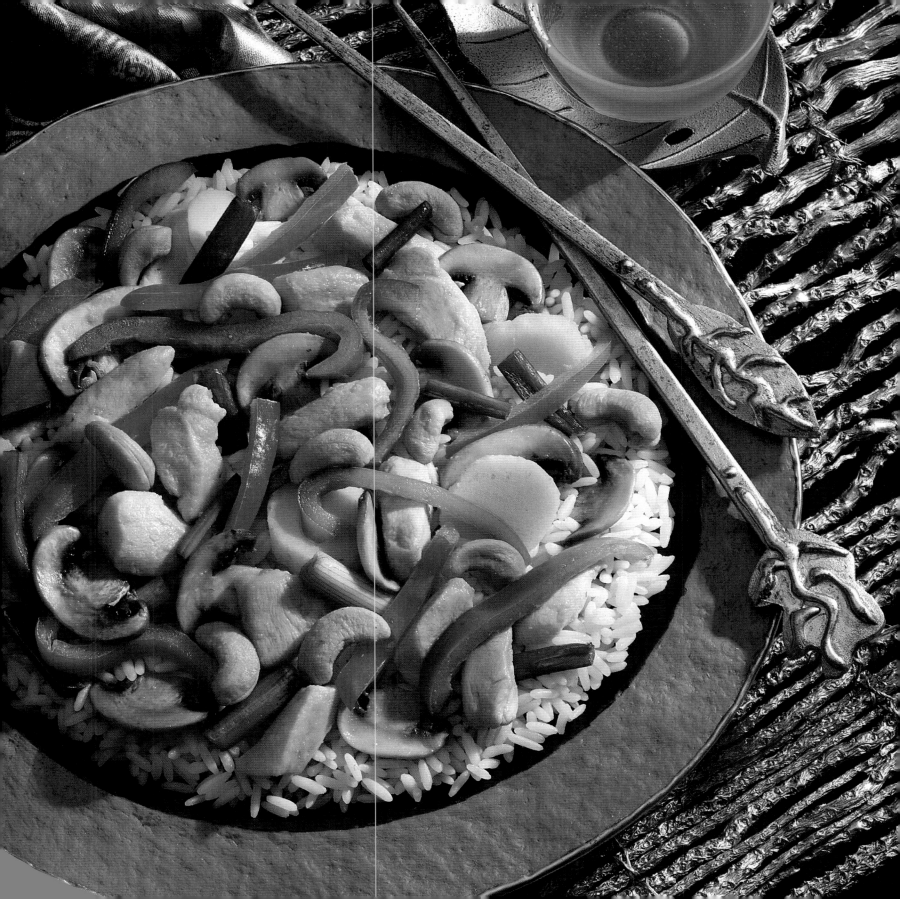

VERSATILE VEGETABLES & SIDES

Pick-of-the-crop vegetables star in this magnificent chapter. Discover your low-fat, high-fiber favorites tucked into scrumptious sides or packed into memorable main dishes.

Green Pea & Rice Almondine

2 teaspoons reduced-calorie margarine
1 cup frozen baby green peas
¼ teaspoon ground cardamom
¼ teaspoon ground cinnamon
Pinch ground cloves
Pinch ground white pepper
¾ cup cooked white rice
2 teaspoons slivered almonds

Melt margarine in medium nonstick skillet over medium heat. Add peas, cardamom, cinnamon, cloves and pepper. Cook and stir 10 minutes or until peas are tender. Add rice. Cook until heated through, stirring occasionally. Sprinkle with almonds before serving.

Makes 4 servings

NUTRIENTS PER SERVING:

Calories	100	Dietary Fiber	2 g
% calories from fat	16	Protein	3 g
Total Fat	2 g	Calcium	19 mg
Saturated Fat	<1 g	Iron	1 mg
Cholesterol	0 mg	Vitamin A	48 RE
Sodium	57 mg	Vitamin C	4 mg
Carbohydrate	18 g		

Dietary Exchanges per Serving: 1 Starch/Bread, ½ Fat

Green Pea & Rice Almondine

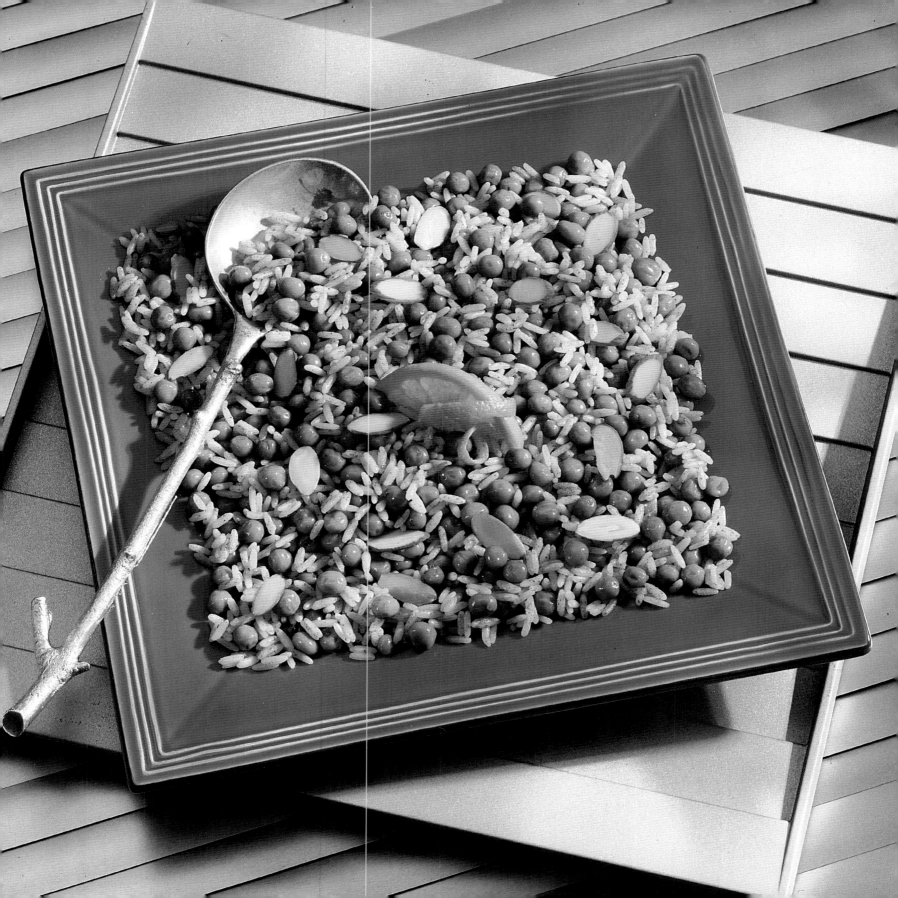

Broccoli with Creamy Lemon Sauce

2 tablespoons fat-free mayonnaise
4½ teaspoons low-fat sour cream
1 tablespoon skim milk
1 to 1½ teaspoons lemon juice
⅛ teaspoon ground turmeric
1¼ cups hot cooked broccoli flowerets

Combine mayonnaise, sour cream, milk, lemon juice and turmeric in top of double boiler. Cook over simmering water 5 minutes or until heated through, stirring constantly. Serve over hot cooked broccoli.

Makes 2 servings

NUTRIENTS PER SERVING:

Calories	44	Dietary Fiber	2 g
% calories from fat	18	Protein	2 g
Total Fat	1 g	Calcium	50 mg
Saturated Fat	<1 g	Iron	1 mg
Cholesterol	4 mg	Vitamin A	132 RE
Sodium	216 mg	Vitamin C	53 mg
Carbohydrate	7 g		

Dietary Exchanges per Serving: 2 Vegetable

Zucchini Cakes

3 teaspoons reduced-calorie margarine, divided
2 tablespoons finely chopped red onion
1 zucchini
½ baking potato, peeled
¼ cup cholesterol-free egg substitute
4½ teaspoons fresh or dry bread crumbs
1 teaspoon chopped dill
Pinch ground white pepper

1. Melt 1½ teaspoons margarine in large skillet. Add onion; cook and stir 5 minutes or until tender.

2. Shred zucchini and potato with grater. Drain. Combine onion, zucchini, potato, egg substitute, bread crumbs, dill and pepper in medium bowl.

3. Melt remaining 1½ teaspoons margarine in large skillet. Drop 4 heaping ¼-cupfuls mixture into skillet; flatten. Cook 10 minutes or until golden brown, turning once. *Makes 2 servings*

NUTRIENTS PER SERVING:

Calories	111	Dietary Fiber	1 g
% calories from fat	24	Protein	5 g
Total Fat	3 g	Calcium	26 mg
Saturated Fat	1 g	Iron	1 mg
Cholesterol	0 mg	Vitamin A	239 RE
Sodium	123 mg	Vitamin C	14 mg
Carbohydrate	17 g		

Dietary Exchanges per Serving: 1 Starch/Bread, ½ Vegetable, ½ Fat

Broccoli with Creamy Lemon Sauce

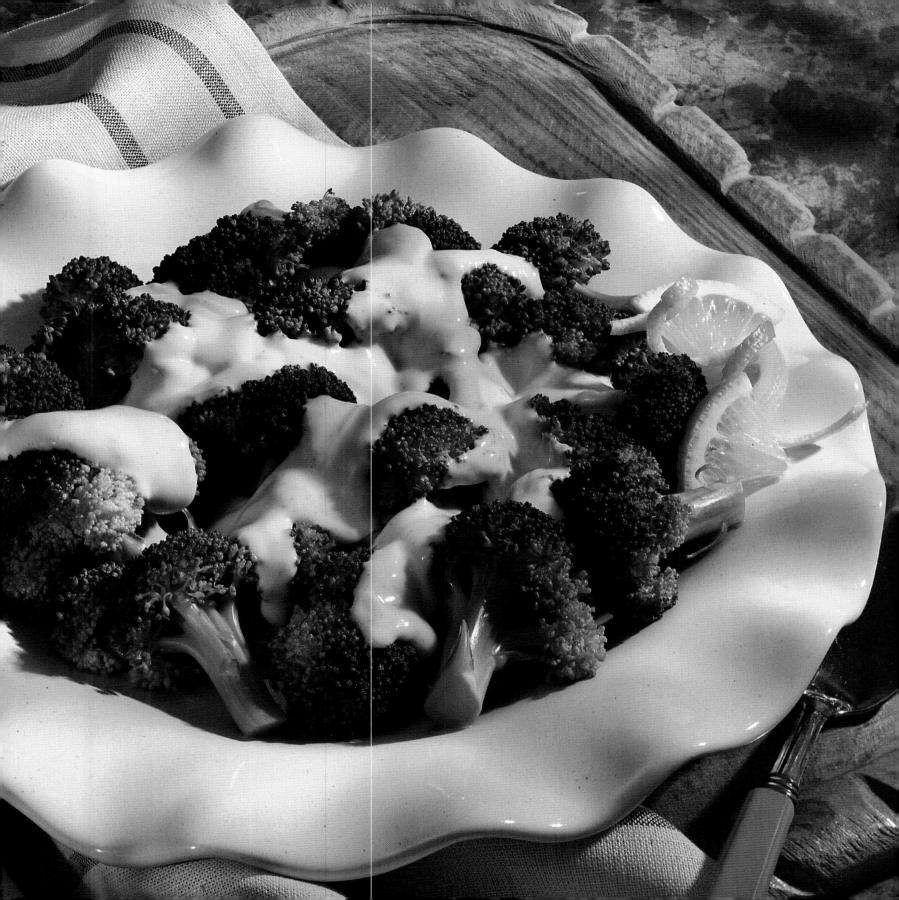

Potatoes au Gratin

1 pound baking potatoes
4 teaspoons reduced-calorie margarine
4 teaspoons all-purpose flour
1¼ cups skim milk
¼ teaspoon ground nutmeg
¼ teaspoon paprika
Pinch ground white pepper
½ cup thinly sliced red onion, divided
⅓ cup fresh or dry whole wheat bread crumbs
1 tablespoon finely chopped red onion
1 tablespoon grated Parmesan cheese

1. Spray 4- or 6-cup casserole with nonstick cooking spray; set aside.

2. Place potatoes in large saucepan; add water to cover. Bring to a boil over high heat. Boil 12 minutes or until potatoes are tender. Drain; let potatoes stand 10 minutes or until cool enough to handle.

3. Melt margarine in small saucepan over medium heat. Add flour. Cook and stir 1 minute or until small clumps form. Gradually whisk in milk. Cook 8 minutes or until sauce thickens, stirring constantly. Remove saucepan from heat. Stir in nutmeg, paprika and pepper.

4. Preheat oven to 350°F. Cut potatoes into thin slices. Arrange half of potato slices in prepared casserole. Sprinkle with half of onion slices. Repeat layers. Spoon sauce over potato mixture. Combine bread crumbs, finely chopped red onion and cheese in small bowl. Sprinkle mixture evenly over sauce.

5. Bake 20 minutes. Let stand 5 minutes before serving. Garnish as desired.   *Makes 4 servings*

NUTRIENTS PER SERVING:

Calories	178	Dietary Fiber	2 g
% calories from fat	14	Protein	6 g
Total Fat	3 g	Calcium	135 mg
Saturated Fat	1 g	Iron	1 mg
Cholesterol	2 mg	Vitamin A	103 RE
Sodium	144 mg	Vitamin C	10 mg
Carbohydrate	33 g		

Dietary Exchanges per Serving: 2 Starch/Bread, ½ Vegetable, ½ Fat

Note: Be sure to read the ingredient list before purchasing whole wheat bread products. The first ingredient listed should be whole wheat flour, not wheat flour. Whole wheat flour contains the wheat germ, which increases the fiber and overall nutritional content of the final product.

Potatoes au Gratin

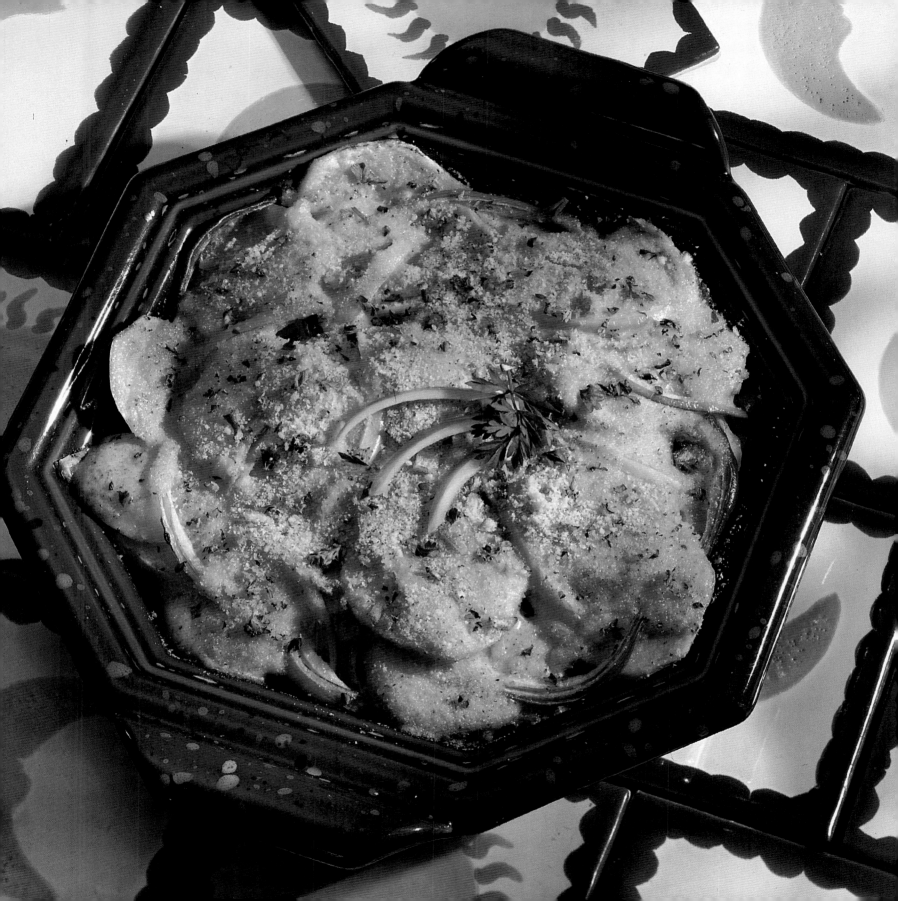

Spiced Mushroom Pecan Rice Timbales

Nonstick cooking spray
1 cup finely chopped shiitake or other mushrooms
¾ cup apple juice
1 (3-inch) cinnamon stick, broken in half
¼ teaspoon salt
3 whole allspice
¾ cup uncooked white basmati rice
¼ cup toasted pecans
3 tablespoons minced fresh chives or green onions

1. Spray 5 (5-ounce) custard cups or molds with cooking spray; set aside.

2. Spray heavy medium saucepan with cooking spray; heat over medium-high heat until hot. Add mushrooms; cook and stir 5 minutes or until tender.

3. Stir ¾ cup water, apple juice, cinnamon sticks, salt and allspice into saucepan; bring to a boil over high heat. Stir in rice; cover. Reduce heat to medium-low. Simmer 15 to 20 minutes or until liquid is absorbed and rice is tender. Remove saucepan from heat. Remove cinnamon sticks and allspice; discard. Stir pecans and chives into saucepan.

4. Spoon rice mixture evenly into prepared cups; pack down with back of spoon. Let stand 5 minutes; unmold onto serving plates. Serve immediately. Garnish as desired.

Makes 5 servings

NUTRIENTS PER SERVING:

Calories	175	Dietary Fiber	1 g
% calories from fat	20	Protein	3 g
Total Fat	4 g	Calcium	10 mg
Saturated Fat	<1 g	Iron	2 mg
Cholesterol	0 mg	Vitamin A	8 RE
Sodium	109 mg	Vitamin C	17 mg
Carbohydrate	33 g		

Dietary Exchanges per Serving: 2 Starch/Bread, ½ Fat

Health Note: Start your search for healthy fare by scouting the front panel of food packages for nutritional claims. Manufacturers that adhere to strict definitions set by the government can advertise information about their products with phrases like Low Fat, Fat Free, Good Source of Calcium and Sodium Free, which makes it easier for consumers to plan healthful meals.

Spiced Mushroom Pecan Rice Timbales

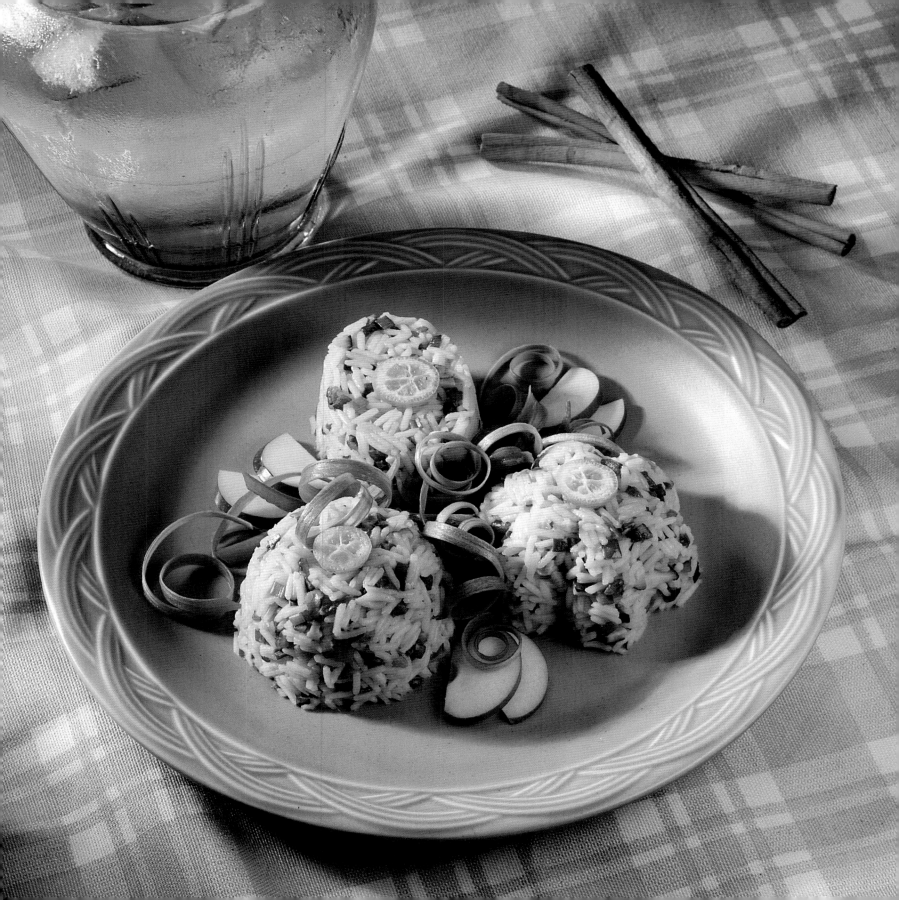

Spaghetti Squash Primavera

2 teaspoons vegetable oil
½ teaspoon finely chopped garlic
¼ cup finely chopped red onion
¼ cup thinly sliced carrot
¼ cup thinly sliced red bell pepper
¼ cup thinly sliced green bell pepper
**1 can (14½ ounces) Italian-style stewed
  tomatoes**
½ cup thinly sliced yellow squash
½ cup thinly sliced zucchini
½ cup frozen whole kernel corn, thawed
½ teaspoon dried oregano leaves
⅛ teaspoon dried thyme leaves
1 spaghetti squash (about 2 pounds)
4 teaspoons grated Parmesan cheese (optional)
2 tablespoons finely chopped fresh parsley

1. Heat oil in large skillet over medium-high heat until hot. Add garlic. Cook and stir 3 minutes. Add onion, carrot and peppers. Cook and stir 3 minutes. Add tomatoes, squash, zucchini, corn, oregano and thyme. Cook 5 minutes or until heated through, stirring occasionally.

2. Cut squash lengthwise in half. Remove seeds. Cover with plastic wrap. Microwave at HIGH 9 minutes or until squash separates easily into strands when tested with fork.

3. Cut each squash half lengthwise in half; separate strands with fork. Spoon vegetables evenly over squash. Top servings evenly with cheese, if desired, and parsley before serving.   *Makes 4 servings*

NUTRIENTS PER SERVING:

Calories	101	Dietary Fiber	5 g
% calories from fat	25	Protein	3 g
Total Fat	3 g	Calcium	70 mg
Saturated Fat	<1 g	Iron	1 mg
Cholesterol	0 mg	Vitamin A	309 RE
Sodium	11 mg	Vitamin C	48 mg
Carbohydrate	18 g		

Dietary Exchanges per Serving: 1 Starch/Bread, 1 Vegetable, ½ Fat

Health Note: Learning to identify high-fat foods items on a menu is an easy way to plan a healthy meal when dining out. Phrases such as broiled, grilled, roasted, stir-fried, and steamed are often used to describe foods that are prepared with less fat. Limit your consumption of foodstuffs that are buttered, basted, fried, or creamed—these food are usually prepared with significant amounts of oil and butter.

Spaghetti Squash Primavera

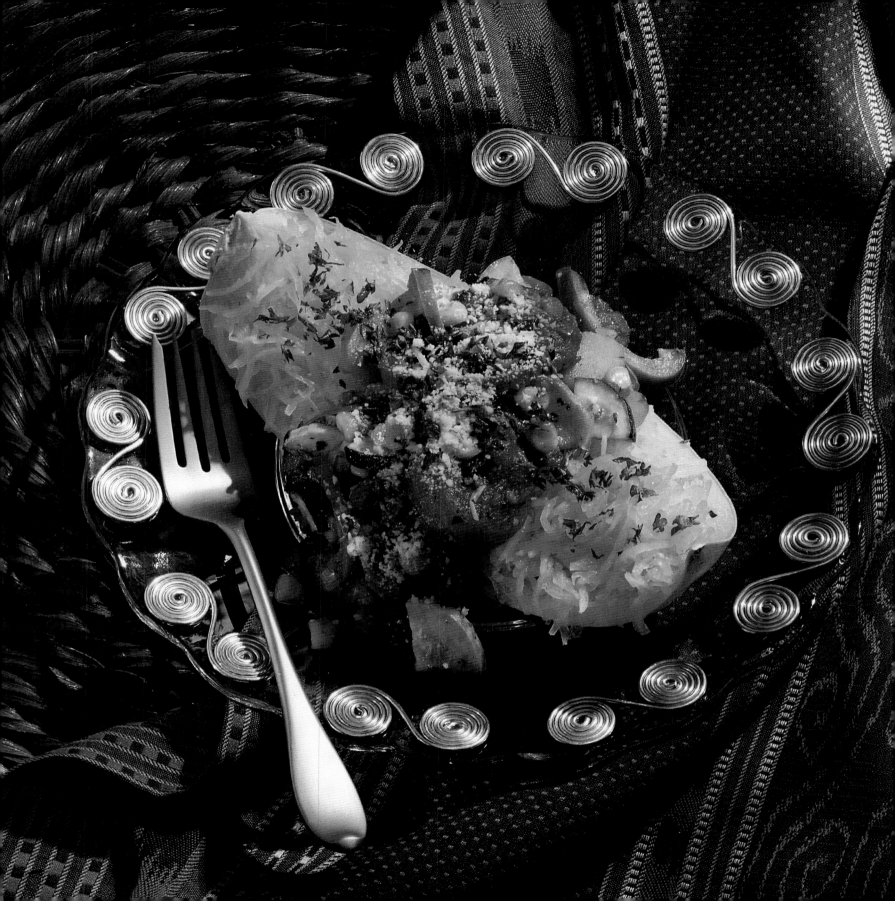

French-Style Green Peas

8 pearl onions
2 small heads Boston lettuce, washed and torn
1½ cups frozen baby green peas, thawed
2 teaspoons finely chopped fresh parsley
⅛ teaspoon dried chervil leaves
    Pinch ground white pepper
1 tablespoon reduced-calorie margarine
½ teaspoon sugar

1. Combine onions and ½ cup water in small saucepan. Bring to a boil over high heat. Reduce heat to medium-high. Simmer 15 minutes or until onions are tender.

2. Add onions, lettuce, peas, parsley, chervil and pepper to saucepan. Bring to a simmer over medium-high heat. Cook 6 minutes or until peas are tender; drain. Stir in margarine and sugar; toss to combine. Serve immediately.   *Makes 2 servings*

NUTRIENTS PER SERVING:

Calories	151	Dietary Fiber	6 g
% calories from fat	20	Protein	8 g
Total Fat	3 g	Calcium	88 mg
Saturated Fat	1 g	Iron	3 mg
Cholesterol	0 mg	Vitamin A	293 RE
Sodium	183 mg	Vitamin C	38 mg
Carbohydrate	24 g		

Dietary Exchanges per Serving: 1½ Starch/Bread, ½ Vegetable, ½ Fat

Corn Soufflé

1 tablespoon reduced-calorie margarine
1 green onion, finely chopped
1 tablespoon all-purpose flour
⅓ cup evaporated skim milk
¾ cup frozen whole kernel corn, thawed
¼ cup cholesterol-free egg substitute
    Pinch ground white pepper
    Pinch ground nutmeg
2 egg whites
½ teaspoon cream of tartar
1 tablespoon grated Parmesan cheese

1. Preheat oven to 375°F. Spray 2-cup soufflé dish with nonstick cooking spray.

2. Melt margarine in medium nonstick skillet over medium heat. Add onion. Cook and stir 2 minutes. Stir in flour. Cook and stir 3 minutes or until small clumps form. Gradually stir in milk with wire whisk. Bring to a boil over high heat, stirring constantly. Combine milk mixture, corn, egg substitute, pepper and nutmeg in medium bowl.

3. With clean beaters, beat egg whites in small bowl with electric mixer at medium speed until soft peaks form. Add cream of tartar. Beat at high speed until stiff peaks form.

4. Gently fold egg whites into corn mixture. Gently spoon mixture into prepared dish. Sprinkle cheese evenly over top of corn mixture.

5. Bake 18 minutes or until knife inserted in center comes out clean. Serve immediately.

Makes 2 servings

NUTRIENTS PER SERVING:

Calories	166	Dietary Fiber	1 g
% calories from fat	21	Protein	12 g
Total Fat	4 g	Calcium	179 mg
Saturated Fat	1 g	Iron	1 mg
Cholesterol	4 mg	Vitamin A	255 RE
Sodium	262 mg	Vitamin C	3 mg
Carbohydrate	22 g		

Dietary Exchanges per Serving: 1 Starch/Bread, 1 Lean Meat, ½ Milk

Spicy Home Fries

2½ teaspoons vegetable oil
1 clove garlic, finely chopped
1 baking potato, peeled
½ teaspoon chili powder
¼ teaspoon ground cumin
¼ teaspoon paprika
⅛ teaspoon ground red pepper
2 tablespoons thinly sliced onion

1. Preheat oven to 350°F. Spray baking sheet with nonstick cooking spray. Combine oil and garlic in small bowl; let stand 15 minutes.

2. Place 1 quart water in medium saucepan; bring to a boil over high heat. Add potato; boil 12 minutes. Drain; let stand 10 minutes or until cool enough to handle. Meanwhile, combine chili powder, cumin, paprika and pepper in small bowl until well blended.*

3. Cut potato into 20 slices. Place onion slices on baking sheet; arrange potato slices on onion. Brush potato slices with half of oil mixture. Sprinkle half of spice mixture over potato slices. Bake 40 minutes, turning once and brushing with remaining oil and spice mixture. *Makes 2 servings*

*Or for mild Home Fries, combine ¼ teaspoon ground paprika, ¼ teaspoon dried oregano leaves, ¼ teaspoon dried thyme leaves, ¼ teaspoon dried sage leaves and ⅛ teaspoon ground red pepper in small bowl until well blended.

NUTRIENTS PER SERVING:

Calories	172	Dietary Fiber	<1 g
% calories from fat	30	Protein	3 g
Total Fat	6 g	Calcium	15 mg
Saturated Fat	<1 g	Iron	1 mg
Cholesterol	0 mg	Vitamin A	39 RE
Sodium	15 mg	Vitamin C	19 mg
Carbohydrate	28 g		

Dietary Exchanges per Serving: 1½ Starch/Bread, 1 Fat

Broccoli & Red Bell Pepper Timbales

2 teaspoons reduced-calorie margarine
¼ cup finely chopped red bell pepper
3 tablespoons finely chopped red onion
⅓ cup cholesterol-free egg substitute
3 tablespoons whole wheat bread crumbs
3 tablespoons nonfat sour cream
2 tablespoons evaporated skim milk
⅛ teaspoon salt
⅛ teaspoon ground nutmeg
Pinch ground black pepper
1 cup cooked frozen chopped broccoli
3 tablespoons shredded reduced-fat Cheddar cheese

1. Preheat oven to 350°F. Spray two 6-ounce custard cups with nonstick cooking spray; set aside.

2. Melt margarine in small saucepan over medium heat. Add bell pepper and onion. Cook and stir 3 minutes or until vegetables are crisp-tender.

3. In food processor or blender combine egg substitute, bread crumbs, sour cream, milk, salt, nutmeg and black pepper; process until well blended. Stir bread crumb mixture, broccoli and cheese into saucepan; blend well.

4. Spoon broccoli mixture evenly into prepared custard cups; pack down with back of spoon. Bake 20 minutes or until mixture is set. Serve in custard cups. *Makes 2 servings*

NUTRIENTS PER SERVING:

Calories	139	Dietary Fiber	5 g
% calories from fat	22	Protein	12 g
Total Fat	4 g	Calcium	225 mg
Saturated Fat	1 g	Iron	2 mg
Cholesterol	6 mg	Vitamin A	714 RE
Sodium	441 mg	Vitamin C	102 mg
Carbohydrate	16 g		

Dietary Exchanges per Serving: 1 Lean Meat, 3 Vegetable

Spinach Parmesan Risotto

3⅔ cups fat-free reduced-sodium chicken broth
½ teaspoon ground white pepper
   Nonstick cooking spray
1 cup uncooked arborio rice
1½ cups chopped fresh spinach
½ cup fresh or frozen green peas
1 tablespoon minced fresh dill or 1 teaspoon
   dried dill weed
½ cup grated Parmesan cheese
1 teaspoon grated lemon peel

1. Combine chicken broth and pepper in medium saucepan; cover. Bring to a simmer over medium-low heat. Keep chicken broth simmering by adjusting heat.

2. Spray large saucepan with cooking spray; heat over medium-low heat until hot. Add rice; cook and stir 1 minute. Stir ⅔ cup hot chicken broth into saucepan; cook, stirring constantly until chicken broth is absorbed.

3. Stir remaining hot chicken broth into rice mixture, ½ cup at a time, stirring constantly until all chicken broth is absorbed before adding next ½ cup. When last ½ cup chicken broth is added, stir spinach, peas and dill into saucepan. Cook, stirring gently until all chicken broth is absorbed and rice is just tender but still firm to the bite. (Total cooking time for chicken broth absorption is about 35 to 40 minutes.)

4. Remove saucepan from heat; stir in cheese and lemon peel. Garnish with lemon slices and fresh dill, if desired.   *Makes 6 servings*

NUTRIENTS PER SERVING:

Calories	179	Dietary Fiber	1 g
% calories from fat	15	Protein	7 g
Total Fat	3 g	Calcium	139 mg
Saturated Fat	2 g	Iron	2 mg
Cholesterol	7 mg	Vitamin A	121 RE
Sodium	198 mg	Vitamin C	6 mg
Carbohydrate	30 g		

Dietary Exchanges per Serving: 2 Starch/Bread,
½ Lean Meat

Health Note: This creamy risotto is packed with calcium and vitamin A. Calcium, which may protect against the development of osteoporosis, may also play a role in the prevention of colon cancer. Vitamin A may prevent the development of cancer as well by boosting the power of the immune system.

Spinach Parmesan Risotto

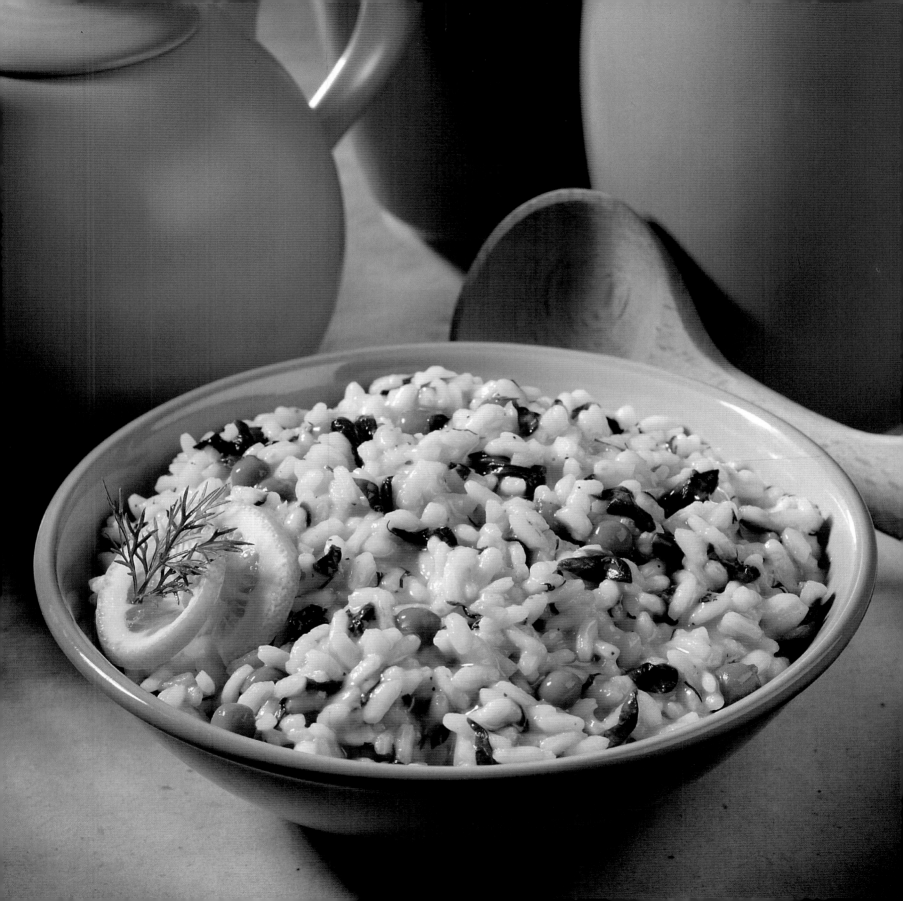

Easy Dilled Succotash

1½ cups frozen lima beans
1 small onion, finely chopped
1½ cups frozen whole kernel corn, thawed
1 teaspoon salt
1 teaspoon sugar
1 teaspoon dried dill weed

1. Bring ½ cup water in medium saucepan to a boil over high heat. Add beans and onion; cover. Reduce heat to low. Simmer 8 minutes.

2. Stir corn into bean mixture; cover. Simmer 5 minutes or until vegetables are tender. Drain bean mixture; discard liquid.

3. Place bean mixture in serving bowl; stir in salt, sugar and dill weed until well blended. Garnish as desired. *Makes 4 servings*

NUTRIENTS PER SERVING:

Calories	126	Dietary Fiber	5 g
% calories from fat	2	Protein	6 g
Total Fat	<1 g	Calcium	28 mg
Saturated Fat	<1 g	Iron	1 mg
Cholesterol	0 mg	Vitamin A	27 RE
Sodium	571 mg	Vitamin C	11 mg
Carbohydrate	28 g		

Dietary Exchanges per Serving: 2 Starch/Bread

Health Note: This simple duo of lima beans and corn has a delightfully upbeat flavor. It's loaded with vitamin E, which along with selenium and other antioxidants, works to neutralize harmful substances, such as smog and cigarette smoke, that have damaging effects on our cells.

Apple-Filled Sweet Potatoes

2 small sweet potatoes or yams
1 Golden Delicious apple, peeled, cored, chopped
5 tablespoons frozen apple juice concentrate, thawed
½ teaspoon ground cinnamon
⅛ teaspoon ground nutmeg

1. Preheat oven to 400°F.

2. Pierce potatoes with fork. Bake 1 hour or until tender. Remove from oven; let stand 10 minutes or until cool enough to handle. Cut potatoes lengthwise in half. Scoop out pulp leaving ¼-inch-thick shells; reserve pulp.

3. Place apple in microwaveable dish; cover with plastic wrap. Microwave at HIGH 90 seconds. Let stand 10 minutes.

4. Preheat broiler. Combine reserved potato pulp, apple juice concentrate, cinnamon and nutmeg in small bowl until well blended. Add apple; toss to coat. Stuff potato halves evenly with apple mixture. Place halves on baking sheet. Broil 5 minutes or until tops are lightly browned. *Makes 4 servings*

NUTRIENTS PER SERVING:

Calories	139	Dietary Fiber	4 g
% calories from fat	2	Protein	2 g
Total Fat	<1 g	Calcium	34 mg
Saturated Fat	<1 g	Iron	1 mg
Cholesterol	0 mg	Vitamin A	2,171 RE
Sodium	12 mg	Vitamin C	36 mg
Carbohydrate	34 g		

Dietary Exchanges per Serving: 1½ Starch/Bread, ½ Fruit

Easy Dilled Succotash

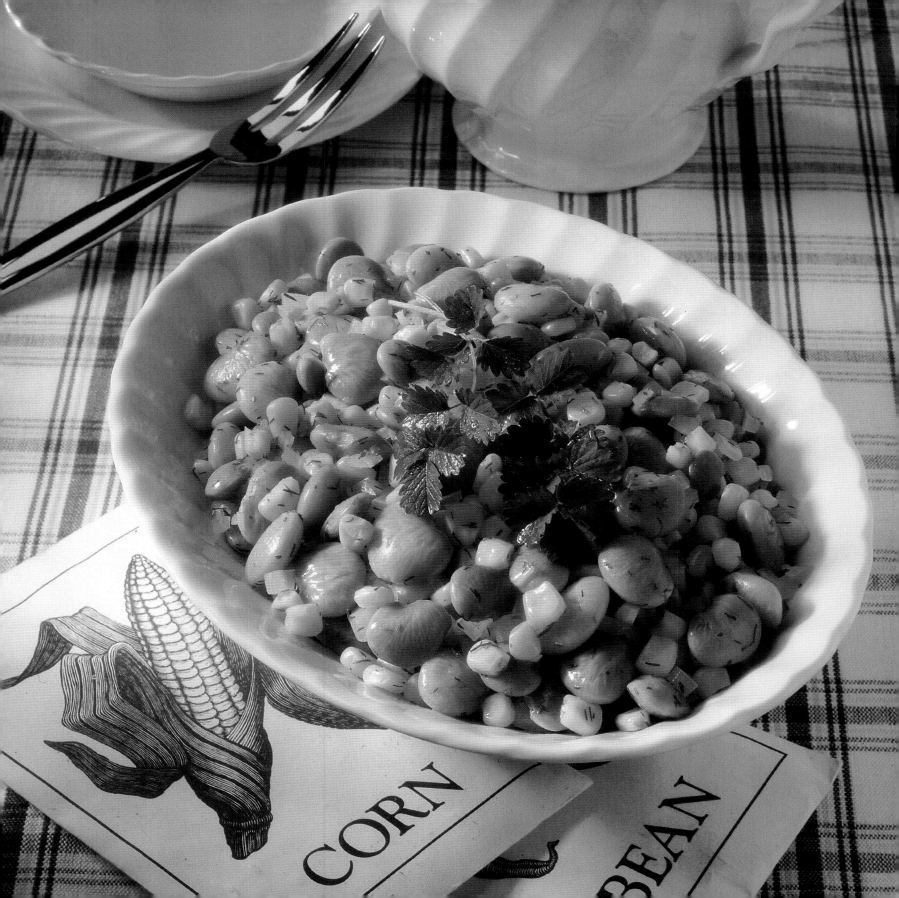

Harvard Beets

2 teaspoons cornstarch
¼ teaspoon salt (optional)
¼ teaspoon grated orange peel
  Ground black pepper
  Dash ground allspice
1 can (16 ounces) sliced beets, drained,
  reserving ⅓ cup liquid
2 tablespoons cider vinegar
1 tablespoon orange juice

1. Microwave Directions: Combine cornstarch, salt, if desired, orange peel, pepper, and allspice in 1-quart microwavable casserole. Blend in reserved beet liquid, vinegar and orange juice.

2. Microwave at HIGH 1¼ to 2½ minutes or until clear and thickened, stirring every minute. Add beets. Microwave at HIGH 2 to 4 minutes or until beets are thoroughly heated.   *Makes 4 servings*

NUTRIENTS PER SERVING:

Calories	42	Dietary Fiber	3 g
% calories from fat	3	Protein	1 g
Total Fat	<1 g	Calcium	18 mg
Saturated Fat	<1 g	Iron	2 mg
Cholesterol	0 mg	Vitamin A	2 RE
Sodium	312 mg	Vitamin C	10 mg
Carbohydrate	10 g		

Dietary Exchanges per Serving: 2 Vegetable

Health Note: Beets are rich in folic acid—a vitamin that is crucial in the normal development of the fetus during pregnancy.

Broccoli & Cauliflower Stir-Fry

2 dry-pack sun-dried tomatoes
4 teaspoons reduced-sodium soy sauce
1 tablespoon rice wine vinegar
1 teaspoon brown sugar
1 teaspoon Oriental sesame oil
⅛ teaspoon crushed red pepper
2¼ teaspoons vegetable oil
2 cups cauliflowerets
2 cups broccoli flowerets
1 clove garlic, finely chopped
⅓ cup thinly sliced red or green bell pepper

1. Place tomatoes in small bowl; cover with boiling water. Let stand 5 minutes. Drain; coarsely chop. Meanwhile, blend soy sauce, vinegar, sugar, sesame oil and red pepper in small bowl.

2. Heat vegetable oil in wok or large nonstick skillet over medium-high heat until hot. Add cauliflower, broccoli and garlic; stir-fry 4 minutes. Add tomatoes and bell pepper; stir-fry 1 minute or until vegetables are crisp-tender. Add soy sauce mixture; cook and stir until heated through. Serve immediately.

Makes 2 servings

NUTRIENTS PER SERVING:

Calories	214	Dietary Fiber	5 g
% calories from fat	30	Protein	9 g
Total Fat	8 g	Calcium	115 mg
Saturated Fat	1 g	Iron	3 mg
Cholesterol	0 mg	Vitamin A	1,493 RE
Sodium	443 mg	Vitamin C	249 mg
Carbohydrate	32 g		

Dietary Exchanges per Serving: 6 Vegetable, 1½ Fat

Harvard Beets

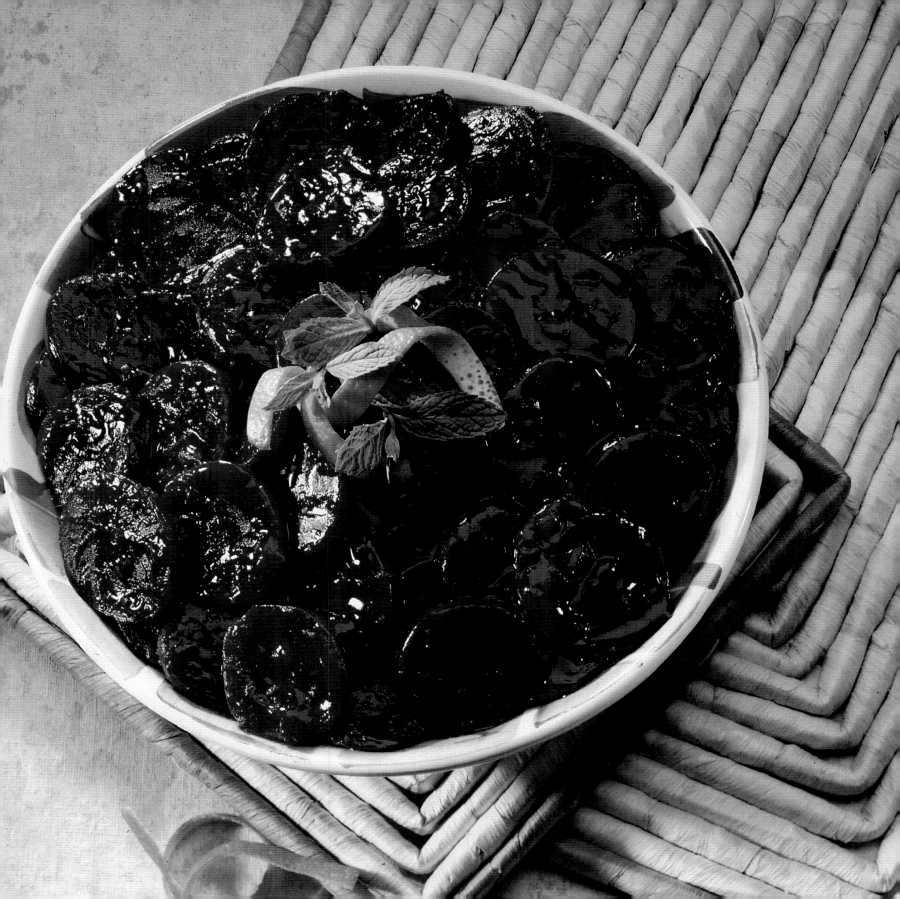

Vegetable Risotto

2 cups broccoli flowerets
1 cup finely chopped zucchini
1 cup finely chopped yellow squash
1 cup finely chopped red bell pepper
2½ cups chicken broth, divided
1 tablespoon extra virgin olive oil
2 tablespoons finely chopped onion
½ cup Arborio or other short-grain rice
¼ cup dry white wine or water
⅓ cup freshly grated Parmesan cheese

1. Steam broccoli, zucchini, yellow squash and bell pepper 3 minutes or just until crisp-tender. Rinse with cold water; drain and set aside.

2. Bring chicken broth to a simmer in small saucepan; keep hot over low heat. Heat oil in heavy, large saucepan over medium-high heat. Add onion to oil; reduce heat to medium. Cook and stir about 5 minutes or until onion is translucent. Add rice, stirring to coat with oil.

3. Add wine; cook and stir until almost dry. Stir ½ cup hot chicken broth into rice mixture; cook until chicken broth is absorbed, stirring constantly. Stir remaining hot chicken broth into rice mixture, ½ cup at a time, stirring constantly until all chicken broth is absorbed before adding next ½ cup. (Total cooking time for chicken broth absorption is about 20 minutes.)

4. Remove saucepan from heat; stir in cheese. Add steamed vegetables; mix well. Serve immediately.

Makes 6 servings

NUTRIENTS PER SERVING:

Calories	150	Dietary Fiber	2 g
% calories from fat	27	Protein	7 g
Total Fat	5 g	Calcium	107 mg
Saturated Fat	1 g	Iron	2 mg
Cholesterol	4 mg	Vitamin A	93 RE
Sodium	253 mg	Vitamin C	59 mg
Carbohydrate	20 g		

Dietary Exchanges per Serving: 1 Starch/Bread, 1 Vegetable, 1 Fat

Braised Oriental Cabbage

½ small head green cabbage (about ½ pound)
1 small head bok choy (about ¾ pound)
½ cup fat-free reduced-sodium chicken broth
2 tablespoons reduced-sodium soy sauce
2 tablespoons rice wine vinegar
1 tablespoon brown sugar
¼ teaspoon crushed red pepper (optional)
1 tablespoon cornstarch
1 tablespoon water

1. Cut cabbage into 1-inch pieces. Cut woody stems from bok choy leaves; slice stems into ½-inch pieces. Cut tops of leaves into ½-inch slices; set aside.

2. Combine cabbage and bok choy stems in large nonstick skillet. Add chicken broth, soy sauce, vinegar, brown sugar and crushed red pepper, if desired.

3. Bring to a boil over high heat. Cover; reduce heat to medium. Simmer 5 minutes or until vegetables are crisp-tender.

4. Blend cornstarch and water in small bowl until smooth. Add to skillet. Cook and stir 1 minute or until sauce boils and thickens.

5. Stir in reserved bok choy leaves; cook 1 minute.

Makes 6 servings

NUTRIENTS PER SERVING:

Calories	34	Dietary Fiber	1 g
% calories from fat	5	Protein	2 g
Total Fat	<1 g	Calcium	67 mg
Saturated Fat	<1 g	Iron	1 mg
Cholesterol	0 mg	Vitamin A	90 RE
Sodium	170 mg	Vitamin C	53 mg
Carbohydrate	6 g		

Dietary Exchanges per Serving: 1½ Vegetable

Vegetable Risotto

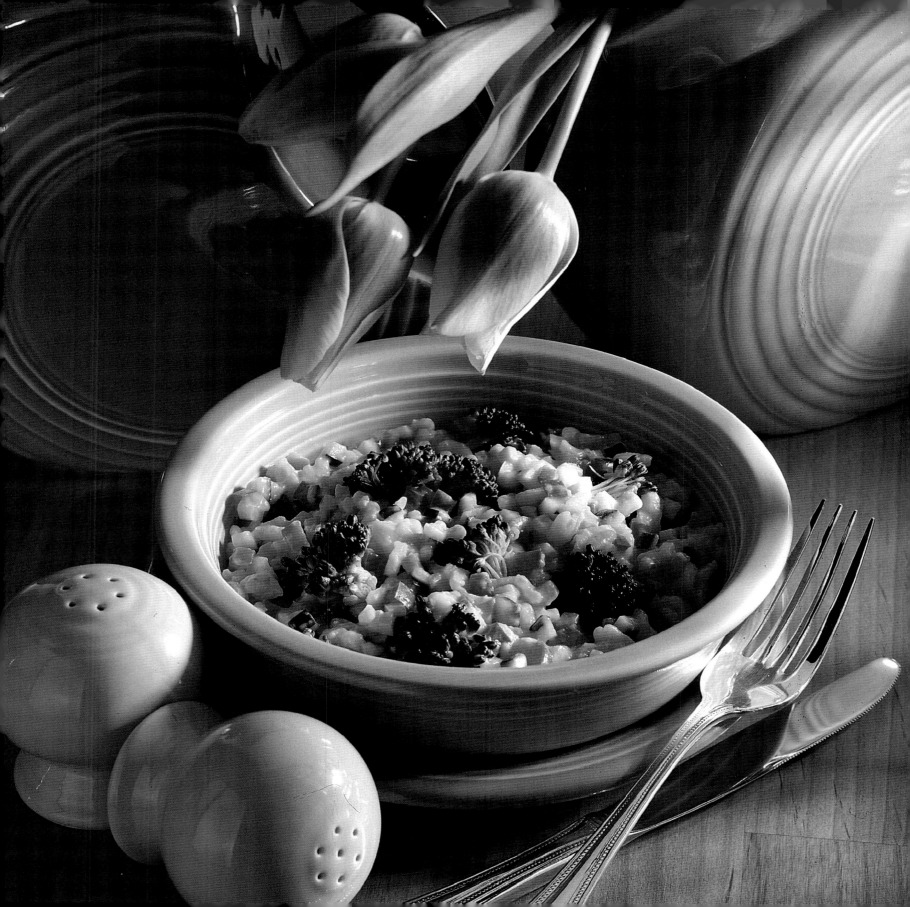

Lemon Broccoli Pasta

Nonstick cooking spray
3 tablespoons sliced green onions
1 clove garlic, minced
2 cups fat-free reduced-sodium chicken broth
1½ teaspoons grated lemon peel
⅛ teaspoon ground black pepper
2 cups frozen or fresh broccoli flowerets
3 ounces uncooked angel hair pasta
⅓ cup low-fat sour cream
2 tablespoons grated Parmesan cheese

1. Generously spray large nonstick saucepan with cooking spray; heat over medium heat until hot. Add green onions and garlic; cook and stir 3 minutes or until onions are tender.

2. Stir chicken broth, lemon peel and pepper into saucepan; bring to a boil over high heat. Add broccoli and pasta; return to a boil. Reduce heat to low. Simmer, uncovered, 6 to 7 minutes, stirring frequently or until pasta is tender.

3. Remove saucepan from heat. Stir in sour cream until well blended. Let stand 5 minutes. Top with cheese before serving. Garnish as desired.

Makes 6 servings

NUTRIENTS PER SERVING:

Calories	100	Dietary Fiber	3 g
% calories from fat	20	Protein	7 g
Total Fat	2 g	Calcium	82 mg
Saturated Fat	<1 g	Iron	1 mg
Cholesterol	6 mg	Vitamin A	186 RE
Sodium	176 mg	Vitamin C	27 mg
Carbohydrate	14 g		

Dietary Exchanges per Serving: ½ Starch/Bread, 1½ Vegetable, ½ Fat

Vegetable-Barley Pilaf

Nonstick cooking spray
¾ cup chopped onion
¾ cup chopped celery
¾ cup sliced fresh mushrooms
¾ cup sliced yellow summer squash
½ cup quick-cooking barley
½ cup sliced carrot
¼ cup chopped fresh parsley
2 teaspoons chopped fresh basil *or* ½ teaspoon dried basil leaves
½ teaspoon chicken-flavor bouillon granules
⅛ teaspoon ground black pepper

1. Coat large skillet with cooking spray. Add onion, celery and mushrooms; cook and stir over medium heat until vegetables are tender.

2. Stir in 1 cup water, squash, barley, carrot, parsley, basil, bouillon granules and pepper. Bring to a boil over high heat. Reduce heat to medium-low. Cover; simmer 10 to 12 minutes or until barley and vegetables are tender.

Makes 4 servings

NUTRIENTS PER SERVING:

Calories	111	Dietary Fiber	5 g
% calories from fat	10	Protein	4 g
Total Fat	1 g	Calcium	37 mg
Saturated Fat	<1 g	Iron	2 mg
Cholesterol	0 mg	Vitamin A	429 RE
Sodium	147 mg	Vitamin C	9 mg
Carbohydrate	22 g		

Dietary Exchanges per Serving: 1 Starch/Bread, 1½ Vegetable

Lemon Broccoli Pasta

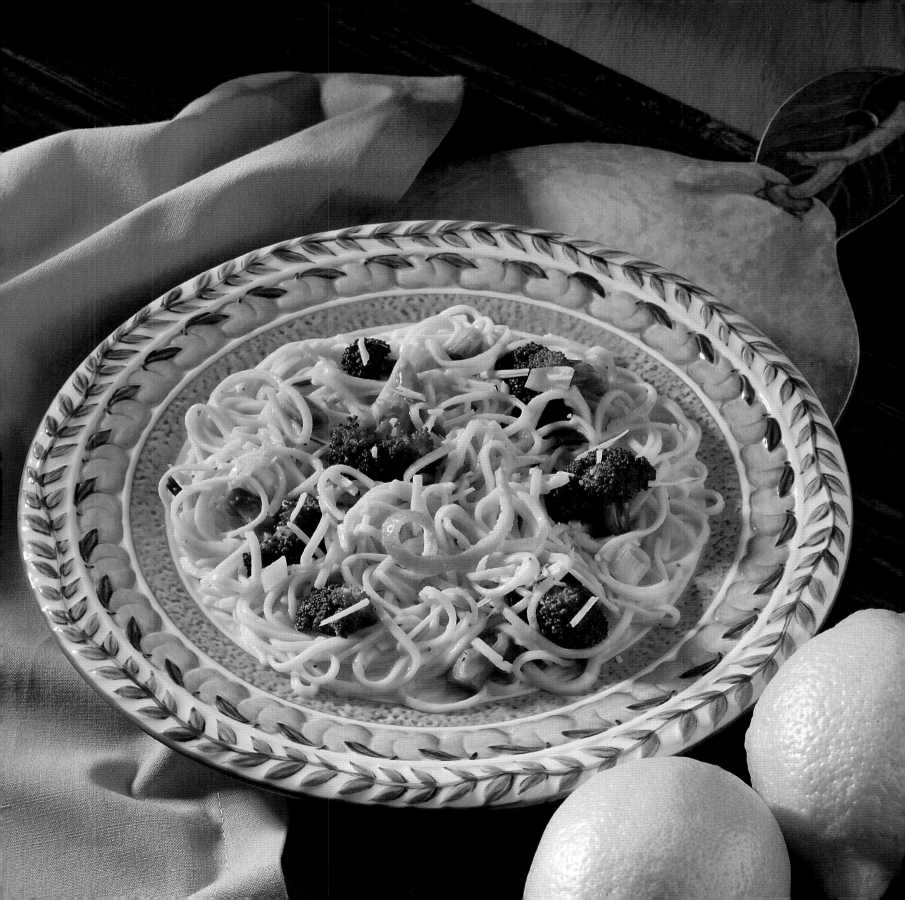

GUILT-FREE DESSERTS

Tickle your taste buds with this dazzling array of luscious, yet lean desserts. Cheesecakes, brownies and cakes have never been so sweet—and so healthy.

Brownie Cake Delight

1 package reduced-fat fudge brownie mix
⅓ cup strawberry all fruit spread
2 cups thawed frozen reduced-fat nondairy whipped topping
¼ teaspoon almond extract
2 cups strawberries, stems removed, halved
¼ cup chocolate sauce

1. Prepare brownies according to package directions, substituting 11×7-inch baking pan. Cool completely in pan.

2. Blend fruit spread and 2 tablespoons water in small bowl until smooth. Combine whipped topping and almond extract in medium bowl.

3. Cut brownie crosswise in half. Place half of brownie, flat-side down, on serving dish. Spread with fruit spread and 1 cup whipped topping. Place second half of brownie, flat-side down, over whipped topping. Spread with remaining whipped topping. Arrange strawberries on whipped topping. Drizzle chocolate sauce onto cake before serving. Garnish with fresh mint, if desired.

Makes 16 servings

NUTRIENTS PER SERVING:

Calories	193	Dietary Fiber	<1 g
% calories from fat	14	Protein	2 g
Total Fat	3 g	Calcium	11 mg
Saturated Fat	<1 g	Iron	1 mg
Cholesterol	<1 mg	Vitamin A	11 RE
Sodium	140 mg	Vitamin C	11 mg
Carbohydrate	41 g		

Dietary Exchanges per Serving: 2 Starch/Bread, ½ Fruit, ½ Fat

Brownie Cake Delight

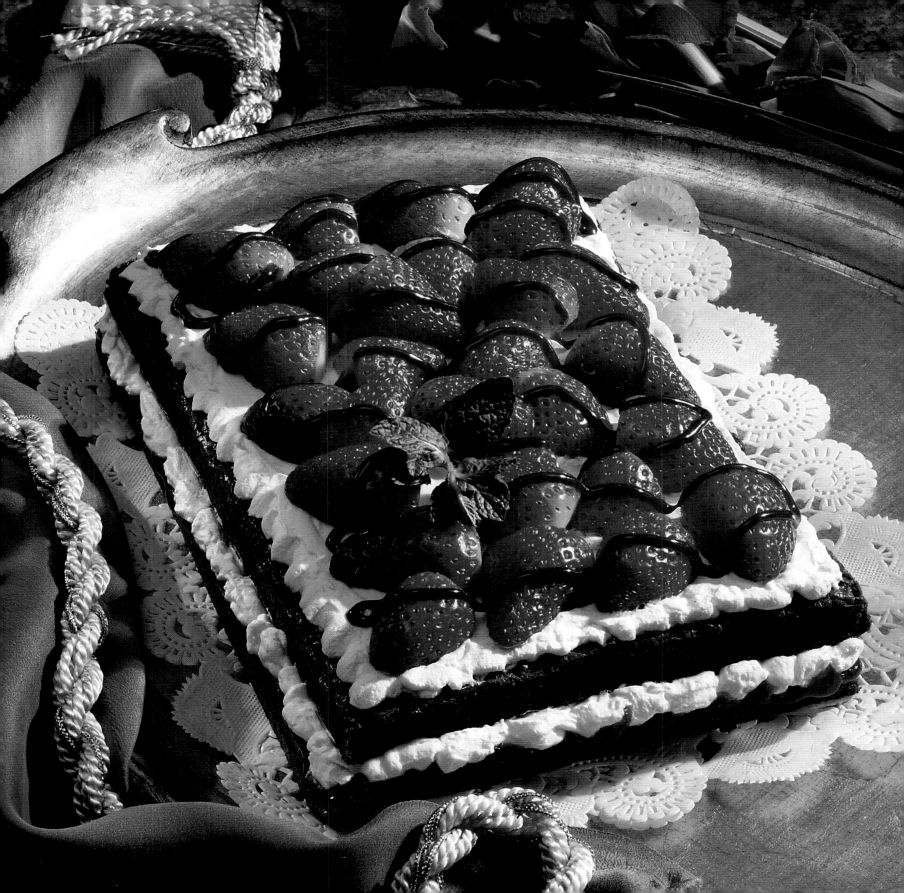

Cheese-Filled Poached Pears

1½ quarts cranberry-raspberry juice cocktail
2 ripe Bartlett pears with stems, peeled
2 tablespoons Neufchâtel cheese
2 teaspoons crumbled Gorgonzola cheese
1 tablespoon chopped walnuts

1. Bring juice to a boil in medium saucepan over high heat. Add pears; reduce heat to medium-low. Simmer 15 minutes or until pears are tender, turning occasionally. Remove pears from saucepan; discard liquid. Let stand 10 minutes or until cool enough to handle.

2. Blend cheeses in small bowl. Cut thin slice off bottom of each pear so that pear stands evenly. Cut pears lengthwise in half, leaving stems intact. Scoop out seeds and membranes to form small hole in each pear half. Fill holes with cheese mixture; press halves together. Place nuts in large bowl; roll pears in nuts. Cover; refrigerate until ready to serve.

Makes 2 servings

NUTRIENTS PER SERVING:

Calories	240	Dietary Fiber	4 g
% calories from fat	24	Protein	4 g
Total Fat	7 g	Calcium	53 mg
Saturated Fat	3 g	Iron	1 mg
Cholesterol	13 mg	Vitamin A	58 RE
Sodium	98 mg	Vitamin C	41 mg
Carbohydrate	45 g		

Dietary Exchanges per Serving: ½ Lean Meat, 3 Fruit, 1 Fat

Health Tip: Start your search for healthy fare by scouting the front panel of food packages for nutritional claims. Manufacturers that adhere to strict definitions set by the government can advertise information about their products with phrases like "Low Fat," "Fat Free," "Good Source of Calcium" and "Sodium Free," which makes it easier for consumers to plan healthful meals.

Mocha Cookies

2 tablespoons plus 1½ teaspoons instant coffee granules
1 tablespoon plus 1½ teaspoons skim milk
⅓ cup packed light brown sugar
¼ cup granulated sugar
¼ cup margarine
1 egg
½ teaspoon almond extract
2 cups all-purpose flour, sifted
¼ cup wheat flake cereal
½ teaspoon ground cinnamon
¼ teaspoon baking powder

1. Preheat oven to 350°F. Spray cookie sheets with nonstick cooking spray.

2. Combine coffee granules and milk in small bowl. Combine sugars and margarine in large bowl with electric mixer. Beat at medium speed until well blended. Beat in egg, almond extract and coffee mixture until smooth.

3. Combine flour, cereal, cinnamon and baking powder in medium bowl. Gradually add to sugar mixture, beating until well blended.

4. Drop teaspoonfuls of dough, 2 inches apart, onto prepared cookie sheets; flatten with back of fork. Bake 8 to 10 minutes or until set. Cool on wire rack.

Makes 3½ dozen cookies

NUTRIENTS PER SERVING: *1 cookie*

Calories	48	Dietary Fiber	<1 g
% calories from fat	25	Protein	1 g
Total Fat	1 g	Calcium	6 mg
Saturated Fat	<1 g	Iron	<1 mg
Cholesterol	5 mg	Vitamin A	19 RE
Sodium	20 mg	Vitamin C	<1 mg
Carbohydrate	8 g		

Dietary Exchanges per Serving: ½ Starch/Bread, ½ Fat

Cheese-Filled Poached Pear

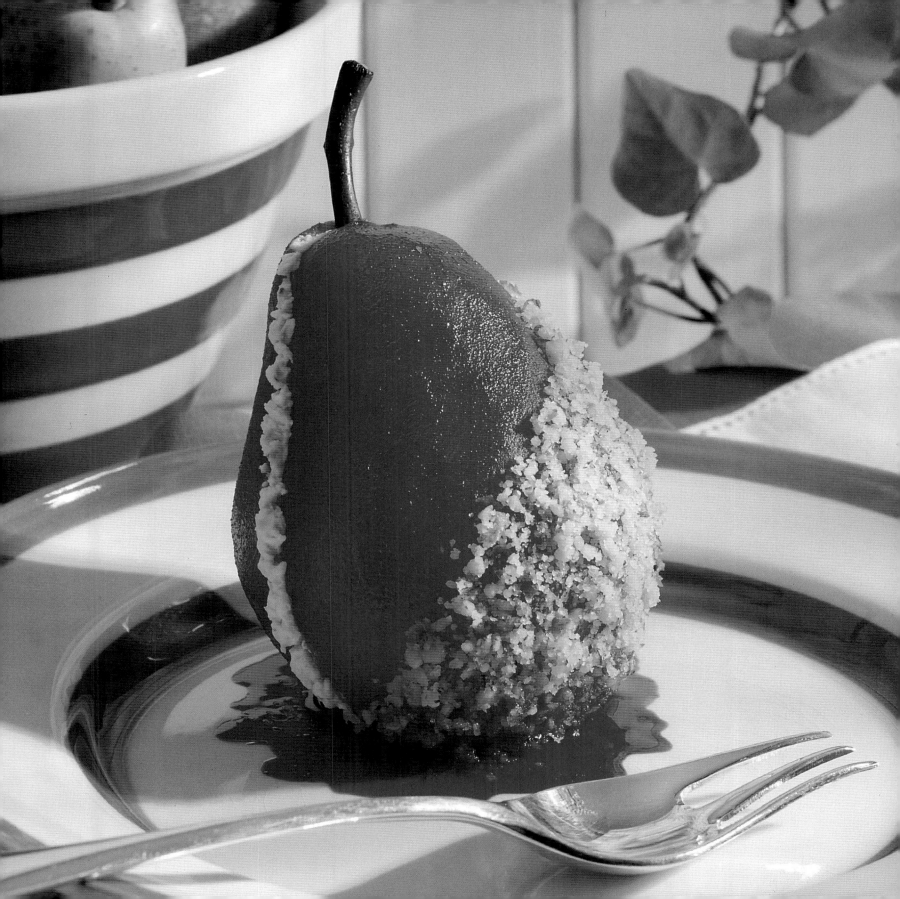

Chocolate-Berry Cheesecake

1 cup chocolate wafer crumbs
1 container (12 ounces) fat-free cream cheese
1 package (8 ounces) reduced-fat cream cheese
⅔ cup sugar
½ cup cholesterol-free egg substitute
3 tablespoons skim milk
1¼ teaspoons vanilla
1 cup mini semisweet chocolate chips
2 tablespoons raspberry all fruit spread
2½ cups fresh strawberries, stems removed, halved

1. Preheat oven to 350°F. Spray bottom of 9-inch springform pan with nonstick cooking spray.

2. Press chocolate wafer crumbs firmly onto side or bottom of prepared pan. Bake 10 minutes. Remove from oven; cool. *Reduce oven temperature to 325°F.*

3. Combine cheeses in large bowl with electric mixer. Beat at medium speed until well blended. Beat in sugar. Beat in egg substitute, milk and vanilla until well blended. Stir in mini chips with spoon. Pour batter into pan.

4. Bake 40 minutes or until center is set. Remove from oven; cool 10 minutes in pan on wire rack. Carefully loosen cheesecake from side of pan. Cool completely.

5. Remove side of pan from cake. Blend fruit spread and 2 tablespoons water in medium bowl until smooth. Add strawberries; toss to coat. Arrange strawberries on top of cake. Refrigerate 1 hour before serving. Garnish with fresh mint, if desired.

Makes 16 servings

NUTRIENTS PER SERVING:

Calories	197	Dietary Fiber	<1 g
% calories from fat	29	Protein	7 g
Total Fat	7 g	Calcium	205 mg
Saturated Fat	2 g	Iron	1 mg
Cholesterol	7 mg	Vitamin A	172 RE
Sodium	290 mg	Vitamin C	13 mg
Carbohydrate	29 g		

Dietary Exchanges per Serving: 1 Starch/Bread, ½ Lean Meat, 1 Fruit, 1 Fat

Cherry Cobbler

1 cup all-purpose flour
¾ cup sugar, divided
2 tablespoons instant nonfat dry milk powder
2 teaspoons baking powder
¼ teaspoon baking soda
¼ teaspoon salt
2 tablespoons vegetable oil
¼ cup plus 3 tablespoons low-fat buttermilk
2 tablespoons cornstarch
½ cup water
1 package (16 ounces) frozen unsweetened cherries, thawed and drained
½ teaspoon vanilla
Fat-free frozen yogurt (optional)

1. Preheat oven to 400°F. Combine flour, ¼ cup sugar, milk powder, baking powder, baking soda and salt in medium bowl. Stir in oil until mixture becomes crumbly. Add buttermilk; stir until moistened. Set aside.

2. Blend cornstarch, remaining ½ cup sugar and water in medium saucepan. Cook over medium heat, stirring constantly, until thickened. Add cherries and vanilla; stir until cherries are completely coated. Pour into 8-inch square baking pan; spoon biscuit mixture over cherries.

3. Bake 25 minutes or until topping is golden brown. Serve warm with fat-free frozen yogurt, if desired.

Makes 8 servings

NUTRIENTS PER SERVING:

Calories	204	Dietary Fiber	1 g
% calories from fat	17	Protein	3 g
Total Fat	4 g	Calcium	53 mg
Saturated Fat	1 g	Iron	1 mg
Cholesterol	1 mg	Vitamin A	58 RE
Sodium	209 mg	Vitamin C	1 mg
Carbohydrate	40 g		

Dietary Exchanges per Serving: 2 Starch/Bread, ½ Fruit, ½ Fat

Cherry Cobbler

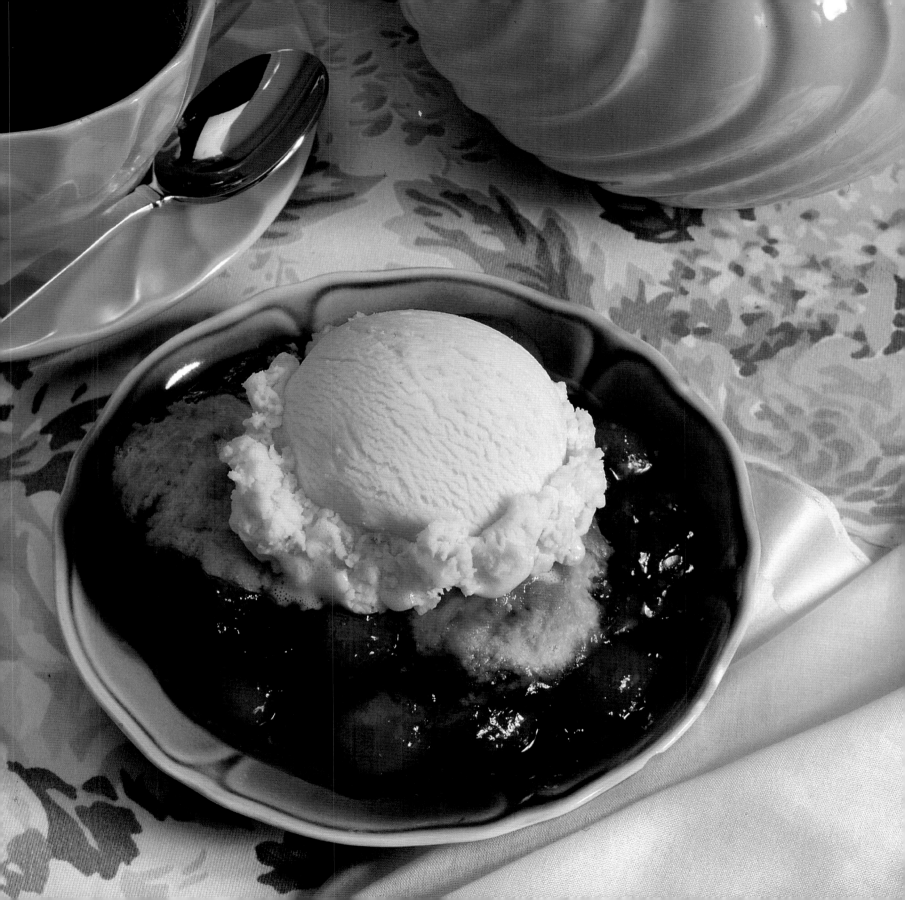

Crème Caramel

½ cup sugar, divided
1 tablespoon hot water
2 cups skim milk
⅛ teaspoon salt
½ cup cholesterol-free egg substitute
½ teaspoon vanilla
⅛ teaspoon maple extract

1. Heat ¼ cup sugar in heavy saucepan over low heat, stirring constantly until sugar is melted and is a light brown color. Remove from heat; stir in hot water. Return to heat; stir 5 minutes or until mixture is a dark caramel color. Divide melted sugar evenly among 6 custard cups. Set aside.

2. Preheat oven to 350°F. Combine milk, remaining ¼ cup sugar and salt in medium bowl. Add egg substitute, vanilla and maple extract; mix well. Pour ½ cup mixture into each custard cup. Place cups in heavy pan; pour hot water into pan to 1- to 2-inch depth.

3. Bake 40 to 45 minutes or until knife inserted near edge of cup comes out clean. Cool on wire rack. Refrigerate at least 4 hours or overnight.

4. When ready to serve, run knife around edge of custard cup. Invert custard onto serving plate; remove cup. _Makes 6 servings_

NUTRIENTS PER SERVING:

Calories	103	Dietary Fiber	0 g
% calories from fat	1	Protein	5 g
Total Fat	<1 g	Calcium	108 mg
Saturated Fat	0 g	Iron	0 mg
Cholesterol	1 mg	Vitamin A	153 RE
Sodium	114 mg	Vitamin C	1 mg
Carbohydrate	21 g		

Dietary Exchanges per Serving: 1 Starch/Bread, ½ Milk

No-Guilt Chocolate Brownies

1 cup semisweet chocolate chips
¼ cup packed brown sugar
2 tablespoons granulated sugar
½ teaspoon baking powder
¼ teaspoon salt
½ cup cholesterol-free egg substitute
1 jar (2½ ounces) first-stage baby food prunes
1 teaspoon vanilla
1 cup uncooked rolled oats
⅓ cup nonfat dry milk solids
¼ cup wheat germ
2 teaspoons powdered sugar

1. Preheat oven to 350°F. Spray 8-inch square baking pan with nonstick cooking spray; set aside. Melt chips in top of double boiler over simmering water.

2. Combine brown and granulated sugars, baking powder and salt in large bowl with electric mixer. Add egg substitute, prunes and vanilla. Beat at medium speed until well blended. Stir in oats, milk solids, wheat germ and chocolate.

3. Pour batter into prepared pan. Bake 30 minutes or until wooden pick inserted in center comes out clean. Cool completely. Cut into 2-inch squares. Dust with powdered sugar before serving. _Makes 16 servings_

NUTRIENTS PER SERVING:

Calories	124	Dietary Fiber	<1 g
% calories from fat	30	Protein	3 g
Total Fat	5 g	Calcium	33 mg
Saturated Fat	<1 g	Iron	1 mg
Cholesterol	<1 mg	Vitamin A	53 RE
Sodium	65 mg	Vitamin C	<1 mg
Carbohydrate	21 g		

Dietary Exchanges per Serving: 1 Starch/Bread, 1 Fat

Crème Caramel

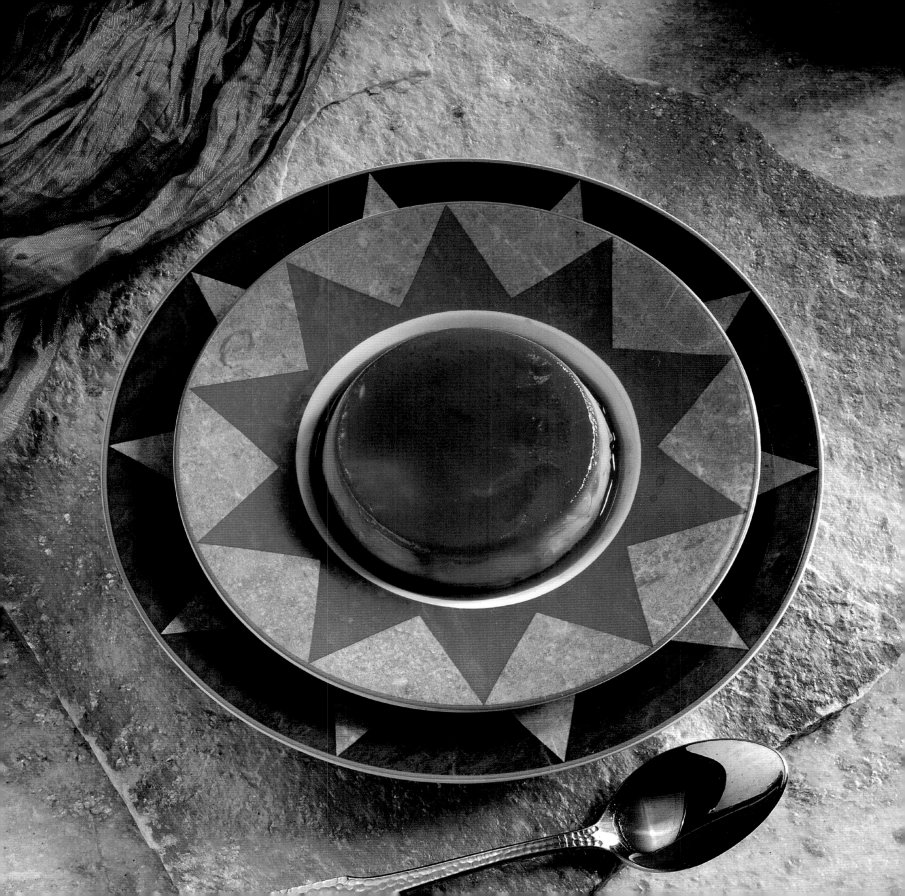

Honey Carrot Cake

   2 cups all-purpose flour
   2 teaspoons baking powder
1½ teaspoons ground cinnamon
   1 cup packed dark brown sugar
   ½ cup honey
   ⅓ cup vegetable oil
   1 egg
   3 egg whites
   3 cups shredded carrots
   1 can (8 ounces) crushed pineapple in juice,
      drained
   ¼ cup chopped toasted pecans
   6 ounces Neufchâtel cheese, softened
   ¾ cup powdered sugar
   1 tablespoon cornstarch
1½ teaspoons vanilla

1. Preheat oven to 350°F. Spray 13×9-inch baking pan with nonstick cooking spray; set aside. Combine flour, baking powder and cinnamon in small bowl; set aside. Beat together brown sugar, honey, oil, egg and egg whites in large bowl with electric mixer. Gradually beat flour mixture into sugar mixture on low speed until well blended. Stir in carrots, pineapple and pecans.

2. Pour batter into prepared pan. Bake 40 to 45 minutes until toothpick inserted in center comes out clean. Cool completely in pan on wire rack.

3. To prepare frosting, blend Neufchâtel cheese, powdered sugar, cornstarch and vanilla in small bowl until smooth. Spread frosting onto top of cake, reserving some frosting to tint with food coloring and pipe into carrot shapes for garnish. Store in refrigerator. *Makes 16 servings*

Variation: Instead of folding pecans into batter, sprinkle pecans over frosted cake.

NUTRIENTS PER SERVING:

Calories	272	Dietary Fiber	1 g
% calories from fat	29	Protein	4 g
Total Fat	9 g	Calcium	42 mg
Saturated Fat	2 g	Iron	1 mg
Cholesterol	22 mg	Vitamin A	623 RE
Sodium	112 mg	Vitamin C	3 mg
Carbohydrate	45 g		

Dietary Exchanges per Serving: 2½ Starch/Bread, ½ Fruit, 1½ Fat

Health Note: The pineapple in this recipe gives the cake a fabulous flavor and also helps to keep it moist without adding fat. In addition, the frosting contains almost no fat since it is made with Neufchâtel cheese, a lighter version of cream cheese.

Honey Carrot Cake

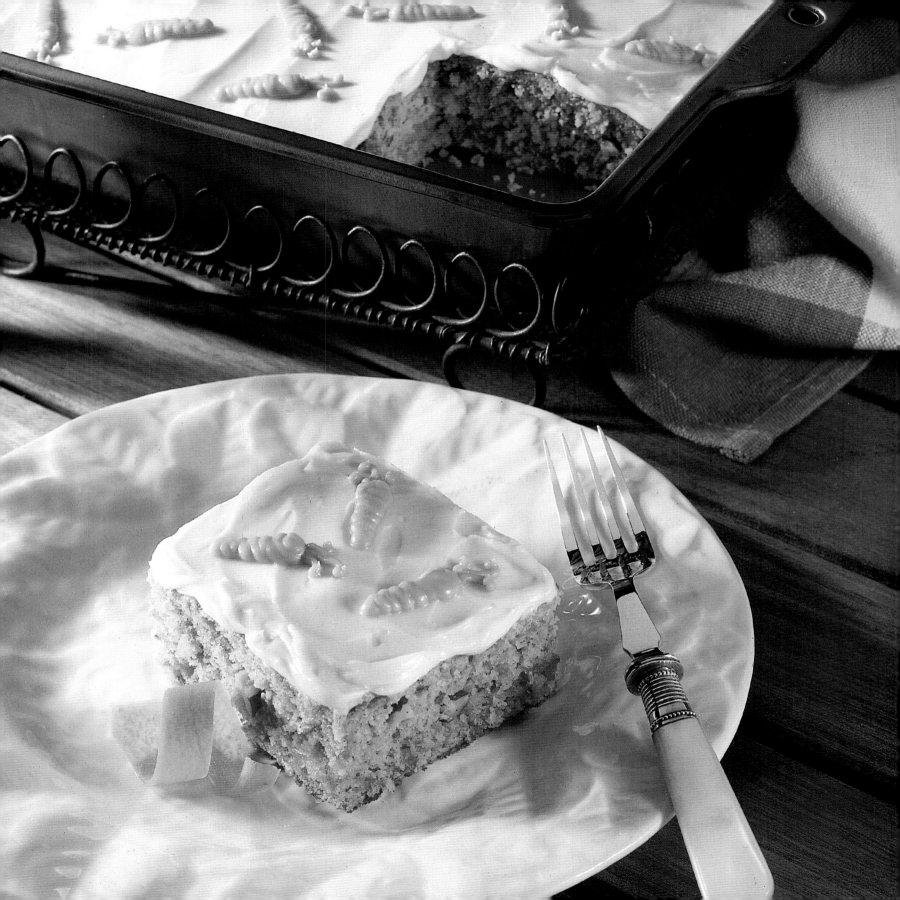

Triple Fruit Trifle

2 ripe pears, peeled, cored, coarsely chopped
2 ripe bananas, thinly sliced
2 cups fresh or thawed frozen raspberries
1 tablespoon lemon juice
¼ cup reduced calorie margarine
1 cup graham cracker crumbs
1 can (12 ounces) evaporated skim milk, divided
⅓ cup sugar
¼ cup cornstarch
⅓ cup cholesterol-free egg substitute
2 tablespoons nonfat sour cream
1½ teaspoons vanilla
3 tablespoons apricot all fruit spread

1. Combine pears, bananas, raspberries and lemon juice in large bowl.

2. Melt margarine in small saucepan over medium heat. Stir in graham cracker crumbs until well blended. Remove saucepan from heat; set aside.

3. Blend ¼ cup milk, sugar and cornstarch in another small saucepan. Whisk in remaining milk. Bring to a boil over medium heat; boil 1 minute or until mixture thickens, stirring constantly. Reduce heat to medium-low.

4. Blend ⅓ cup hot milk mixture and egg substitute in small bowl. Add to milk mixture. Cook 2 minutes, stirring constantly. Remove saucepan from heat. Let stand 10 minutes, stirring frequently. Stir in sour cream and vanilla; blend well.

5. Spoon half of milk mixture into trifle dish or medium straight-sided glass serving bowl. Layer half of fruit mixture and ½ cup graham cracker crumb mixture over milk mixture. Repeat layers, ending with graham cracker crumb mixture. Blend fruit spread and 1 teaspoon water until smooth. Drizzle over trifle. Garnish with additional fresh fruit, if desired.

Makes 12 servings

NUTRIENTS PER SERVING:

Calories	181	Dietary Fiber	2 g
% calories from fat	17	Protein	5 g
Total Fat	3 g	Calcium	124 mg
Saturated Fat	<1 g	Iron	1 mg
Cholesterol	1 mg	Vitamin A	135 RE
Sodium	151 mg	Vitamin C	9 mg
Carbohydrate	34 g		

Dietary Exchanges per Serving: ½ Starch/Bread, ½ Milk, 1½ Fruit, ½ Fat

Nectarine Meringue Crowns

2 egg whites
⅛ teaspoon cream of tartar
⅛ teaspoon ground nutmeg
⅔ cup sugar
1 can (6 ounces) frozen cranberry juice concentrate, thawed
1 tablespoon plus 1½ teaspoons cornstarch
5 fresh nectarines, halved, pitted and sliced

1. Preheat oven to 250°F. Beat egg whites, cream of tartar and nutmeg in small bowl with electric mixer at medium speed until foamy. Gradually add sugar, beating until stiff peaks form. Divide meringue into 6 equal mounds on baking sheet; shape into round tarts. Bake 1 hour; cool.

2. Pour cranberry juice concentrate into medium saucepan. Stir in ½ cup water and cornstarch. Cook, stirring constantly, until sauce thickens; cool. Fill each meringue tart with about ½ cup nectarine slices; drizzle with sauce.

Makes 6 servings

NUTRIENTS PER SERVING:

Calories	203	Dietary Fiber	2 g
% calories from fat	2	Protein	2 g
Total Fat	1 g	Calcium	10 mg
Saturated Fat	<1 g	Iron	<1 mg
Cholesterol	0 mg	Vitamin A	84 RE
Sodium	20 mg	Vitamin C	28 mg
Carbohydrate	50 g		

Dietary Exchanges per Serving: 3½ Fruit

Triple Fruit Trifle

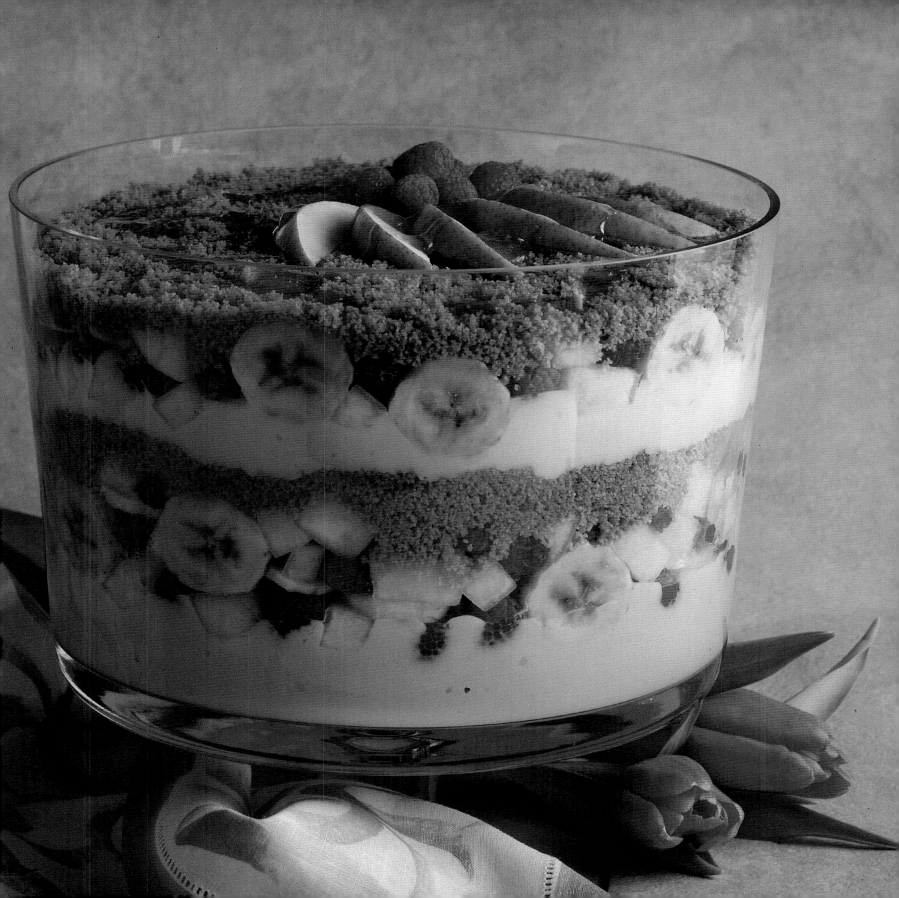

Turtle Cheesecake

6 tablespoons reduced-calorie margarine
1½ cups graham cracker crumbs
2 envelopes unflavored gelatin
2 containers (8 ounces each) fat-free cream cheese
2 cups 1% low fat cottage cheese
1 cup sugar
1½ teaspoons vanilla
1 container (8 ounces) frozen reduced-fat nondairy whipped topping, thawed
¼ cup prepared fat-free caramel topping
¼ cup prepared fat-free hot fudge topping
¼ cup chopped pecans

1. Spray bottom and side of 9-inch springform pan with nonstick cooking spray. Preheat oven to 350°F. Melt margarine in small saucepan over medium heat. Stir in graham cracker crumbs. Press crumb mixture firmly onto side or bottom of prepared pan. Bake 10 minutes. Cool.

2. Place ½ cup cold water in small saucepan; sprinkle gelatin over water. Let stand 3 minutes to soften. Heat gelatin mixture over low heat until completely dissolved, stirring constantly.

3. Combine cream cheese, cottage cheese, sugar and vanilla in food processor or blender; process until smooth. Add gelatin mixture; process until well blended. Fold in whipped topping. Pour into prepared crust. Refrigerate 4 hours or until set.

4. Loosen cake from side of pan. Remove side of pan from cake. Drizzle caramel and hot fudge toppings over cheesecake. Sprinkle pecans evenly over top of cake before serving. *Makes 16 servings*

NUTRIENTS PER SERVING:

Calories	232	Dietary Fiber	<1 g
% calories from fat	26	Protein	10 g
Total Fat	7 g	Calcium	240 mg
Saturated Fat	1 g	Iron	1 mg
Cholesterol	5 mg	Vitamin A	164 RE
Sodium	444 mg	Vitamin C	1 mg
Carbohydrate	32 g		

Dietary Exchanges per Serving: 2 Starch/Bread, ½ Lean Meat, 1 Fat

Health Note: A meal plan high in dietary calcium may actually protect—not cause—the formation of kidney stones. Studies indicate that calcium, abundant in foods like milk, yogurt, cottage cheese and ricotta cheese, appears to bind oxalates which are linked to the formation of the stones.

Turtle Cheesecake

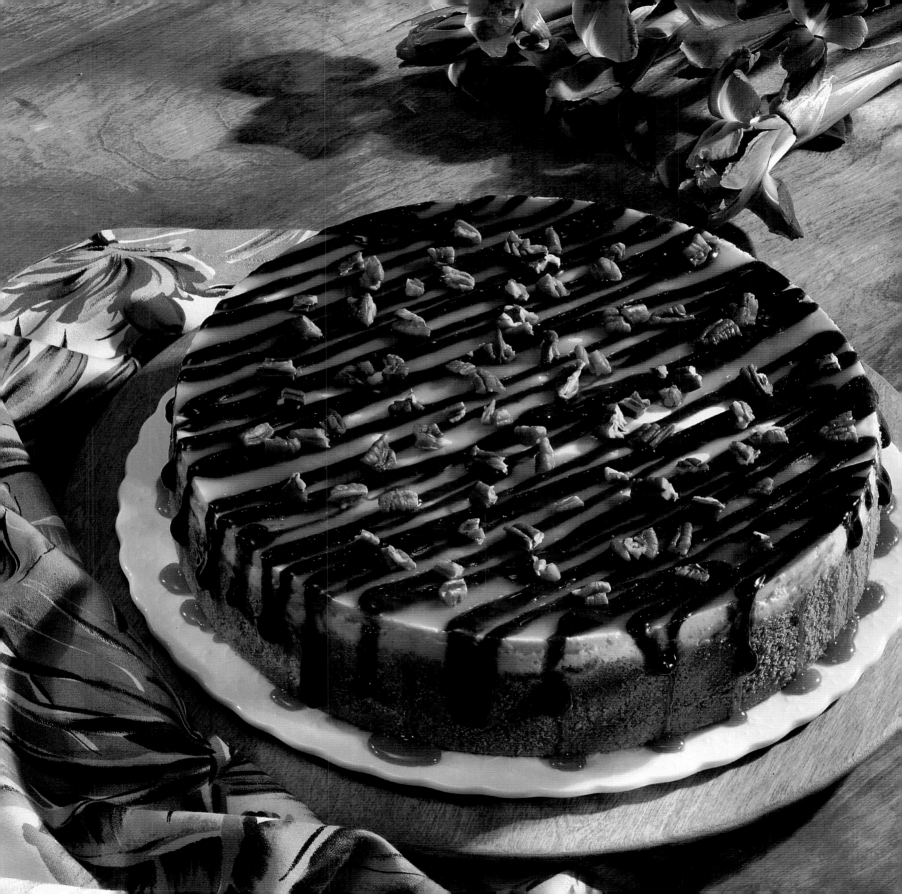

Blueberry Chiffon Cake

3 tablespoons reduced-calorie margarine
¾ cup graham cracker crumbs
2 cups fresh or thawed frozen blueberries
2 envelopes unflavored gelatin
2 containers (8 ounces each) fat-free cream cheese
1 container (8 ounces) Neufchâtel cheese
¾ cup sugar, divided
⅔ cup nonfat sour cream
½ cup lemon juice
1 tablespoon grated lemon peel
6 egg whites*

*Use only grade A clean, uncracked eggs.

1. Preheat oven to 350°F.

2. Melt margarine in small saucepan over medium heat. Stir in graham cracker crumbs. Press crumb mixture firmly onto bottom and 1 inch up side of 9-inch springform pan. Bake 10 minutes. Remove from oven. Cool 10 minutes. Arrange blueberries in a single layer on top of crust. Refrigerate until needed.

3. Place ½ cup cold water in small saucepan; sprinkle gelatin over water. Let stand 3 minutes to soften. Heat gelatin mixture over low heat until completely dissolved, stirring constantly.

4. Combine cheeses in large bowl with electric mixer. Beat at medium speed until well blended. Beat in ½ cup sugar until well blended. Beat in sour cream, lemon juice and lemon peel until well blended. Beat in gelatin mixture until well blended.

5. With clean, dry beaters, beat egg whites in medium bowl with electric mixer at medium speed until soft peaks form. Gradually add remaining ¼ cup sugar. Beat at high speed until stiff peaks form. Fold egg whites into cream cheese mixture. Gently spoon mixture into prepared crust. Cover with plastic wrap. Refrigerate 6 hours or until set.   *Makes 16 servings*

NUTRIENTS PER SERVING:

Calories	165	Dietary Fiber	1 g
% calories from fat	28	Protein	10 g
Total Fat	5 g	Calcium	229 mg
Saturated Fat	2 g	Iron	0 mg
Cholesterol	14 mg	Vitamin A	203 RE
Sodium	342 mg	Vitamin C	6 mg
Carbohydrate	20 g		

Dietary Exchanges per Serving: ½ Starch/Bread, 1 Lean Meat, 1 Fruit, ½ Fat

Chocolate Angel Fruit Torte

1 package chocolate angel food cake mix
2 bananas, thinly sliced
1½ teaspoons lemon juice
1 can (12 ounces) evaporated skim milk, divided
⅓ cup sugar
¼ cup cornstarch
⅓ cup cholesterol-free egg substitute
3 tablespoons nonfat sour cream
3 teaspoons vanilla
3 large kiwis, peeled, thinly sliced
1 can (11 ounces) mandarin orange segments, rinsed, drained

1. Prepare cake according to package directions; cool completely. Cut horizontally in half to form 2 layers; set aside.

2. Place banana slices in medium bowl. Add lemon juice; toss to coat. Set aside.

3. Combine ¼ cup milk, sugar and cornstarch in small saucepan; whisk until smooth. Whisk in remaining milk. Bring to a boil over high heat, stirring constantly. Boil 1 minute or until mixture thickens, stirring constantly. Reduce heat to medium-low.

4. Blend ⅓ cup hot milk mixture and egg substitute in small bowl. Add to saucepan. Cook 2 minutes, stirring constantly. Remove saucepan from heat. Let stand 10 minutes, stirring frequently. Add sour cream and vanilla; blend well.

5. Place bottom half of cake on serving plate. Spread with half of milk mixture. Arrange half of banana slices, kiwi slices and mandarin orange segments on milk mixture. Place remaining half of cake, cut-side down, over fruit. Top with remaining milk mixture and fruit. Refrigerate until ready to serve.

Makes 12 servings

NUTRIENTS PER SERVING:

Calories	233	Dietary Fiber	1 g
% calories from fat	1	Protein	7 g
Total Fat	<1 g	Calcium	150 mg
Saturated Fat	<1 g	Iron	1 mg
Cholesterol	1 mg	Vitamin A	113 RE
Sodium	306 mg	Vitamin C	30 mg
Carbohydrate	52 g		

Dietary Exchanges per Serving: 2½ Starch/Bread, 1 Fruit

Cook's Tip: Angel food cakes need to be inverted during cooling to prevent them from falling. An easy way to invert your cake is to position the tube over a narrow-necked bottle.

Cheesy Cherry Turnovers

Butter-flavored nonstick cooking spray
1 package (8 ounces) reduced-fat cream cheese, softened
1 cup 1% low-fat cottage cheese
½ cup sugar, divided
1 teaspoon vanilla
1 can (16½ ounces) dark sweet pitted cherries, rinsed and drained
8 sheets frozen phyllo dough, thawed
1 cup whole wheat bread crumbs
1 teaspoon ground cinnamon

1. Preheat oven to 350°F. Spray baking sheet with cooking spray; set aside.

2. Combine cream cheese, cottage cheese, ¼ cup sugar and vanilla in medium bowl with electric mixer. Beat at medium speed until well blended. Stir in cherries.

3. Spray 1 phyllo dough sheet with cooking spray; fold sheet crosswise in half to form rectangle. Sprinkle with 2 tablespoons bread crumbs. Drop ⅓ cup cheese mixture onto upper left corner of sheet. Fold left corner over mixture to form triangle. Continue folding triangle, right to left, until end of dough. Repeat with remaining ingredients. Place turnovers on prepared baking sheet. Combine remaining ¼ cup sugar with cinnamon. Sprinkle turnovers with sugar mixture.

4. Bake 12 to 15 minutes or until turnovers are crisp and golden brown. Serve warm or cold.

Makes 8 servings

NUTRIENTS PER SERVING:

Calories	170	Dietary Fiber	1 g
% calories from fat	29	Protein	8 g
Total Fat	6 g	Calcium	74 mg
Saturated Fat	3 g	Iron	1 mg
Cholesterol	11 mg	Vitamin A	170 RE
Sodium	314 mg	Vitamin C	1 mg
Carbohydrate	24 g		

Dietary Exchanges per Serving: 1 Starch/Bread, ½ Lean Meat, ½ Fruit, 1 Fat

Peach & Blackberry Shortcakes

¾ **cup plain low-fat yogurt, divided**
5 **teaspoons sugar, divided**
1 **tablespoon blackberry all fruit spread**
½ **cup coarsely chopped peeled peach**
½ **cup fresh or thawed frozen blackberries or**
   raspberries
½ **cup all-purpose flour**
¼ **teaspoon baking powder**
⅛ **teaspoon baking soda**
2 **tablespoons reduced-calorie margarine**
½ **teaspoon vanilla**

1. Place cheesecloth or coffee filter in large sieve or strainer. Spoon yogurt into sieve; place over large bowl. Refrigerate 20 minutes. Remove yogurt from sieve; discard liquid. Measure ¼ cup yogurt; blend remaining ½ cup yogurt, 2 teaspoons sugar and fruit spread in small bowl. Refrigerate until ready to serve.

2. Meanwhile, combine peach, blackberries and ½ teaspoon sugar in medium bowl; set aside.

3. Preheat oven to 425°F. Combine flour, baking powder, baking soda and remaining 2½ teaspoons sugar in small bowl. Cut in margarine with pastry blender until mixture resembles coarse crumbs. Combine reserved ¼ cup yogurt with vanilla. Stir into flour mixture just until dry ingredients are moistened. Shape dough into a ball.

4. Place dough on lightly floured surface. Knead dough gently 8 times. Divide dough in half. Roll out each half into 3-inch circle with lightly floured rolling pin. Place circles on ungreased baking sheet.

5. Bake 12 to 15 minutes or until lightly browned. Immediately remove from baking sheet. Cool shortcakes on wire rack 10 minutes or until cool enough to handle.

6. Cut shortcakes in half. Top bottom halves with fruit and yogurt mixtures and remaining halves. Garnish with blackberries and mint, if desired. Serve immediately.

Makes 2 servings

NUTRIENTS PER SERVING:

Calories	327	Dietary Fiber	4 g
% calories from fat	21	Protein	8 g
Total Fat	8 g	Calcium	183 mg
Saturated Fat	2 g	Iron	2 mg
Cholesterol	5 mg	Vitamin A	176 RE
Sodium	311 mg	Vitamin C	11 mg
Carbohydrate	57 g		

Dietary Exchanges per Serving: 2½ Starch/Bread,
½ Milk, 1 Fruit, 1 Fat

Peach & Blackberry Shortcake

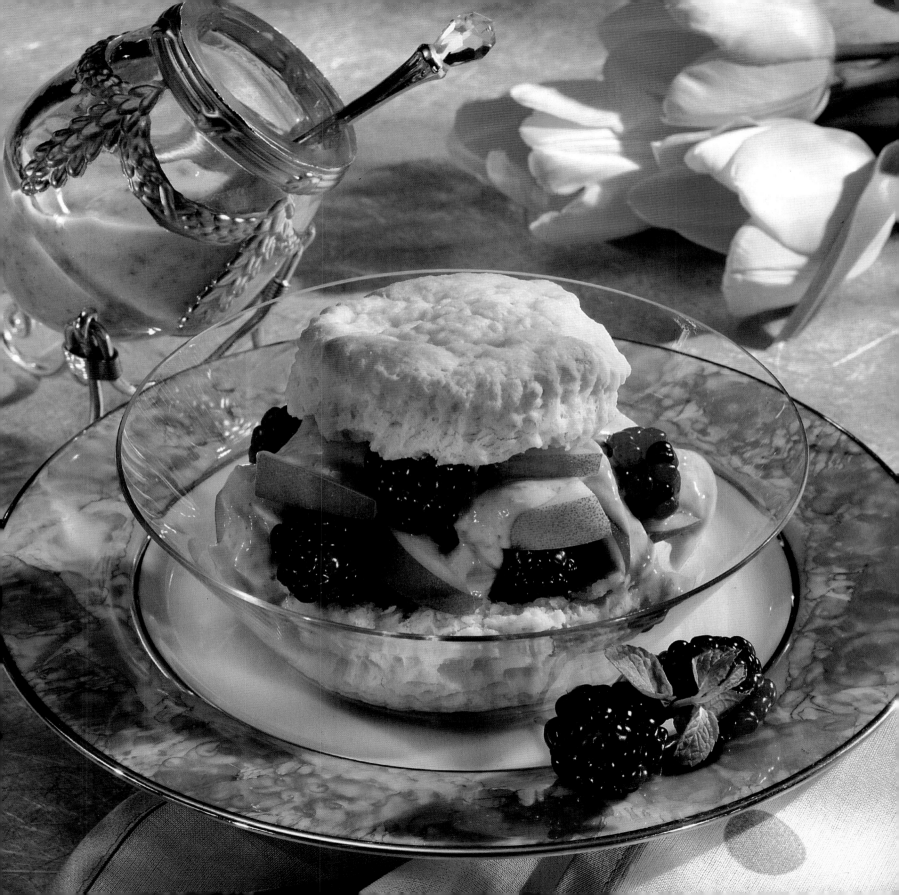

Mocha Crinkles

1⅓ cups packed light brown sugar
½ cup vegetable oil
¼ cup low-fat sour cream
1 egg
1 teaspoon vanilla
1¾ cups all-purpose flour
¾ cup unsweetened cocoa powder
2 teaspoons instant espresso or coffee
   granules
1 teaspoon baking soda
¼ teaspoon salt
⅛ teaspoon ground black pepper
½ cup powdered sugar

1. Combine brown sugar and oil in medium bowl with electric mixer. Beat at medium speed until well blended. Beat in sour cream, egg and vanilla.

2. Mix flour, cocoa, espresso, baking soda, salt and pepper in another medium bowl.

3. Beat in flour mixture until soft dough forms. Form dough into disc; cover. Refrigerate dough until firm, 3 to 4 hours.

4. Preheat oven to 350°F. Place powdered sugar in shallow bowl. Cut dough into 1-inch pieces; roll into balls. Coat with powdered sugar. Place on ungreased cookie sheets.

5. Bake 10 to 12 minutes or until tops of cookies are firm to the touch. *Do not overbake.* Cool completely on wire racks. *Makes 6 dozen cookies*

NUTRIENTS PER SERVING: *1 cookie*

Calories	44	Dietary Fiber	0 g
% calories from fat	30	Protein	0 g
Total Fat	1 g	Calcium	7 mg
Saturated Fat	<1 g	Iron	1 mg
Cholesterol	3 mg	Vitamin A	4 RE
Sodium	28 mg	Vitamin C	0 mg
Carbohydrate	7 g		

Dietary Exchanges per Serving: ½ Starch/Bread

Blackberry Strudel Cups

6 sheets frozen phyllo dough, thawed
   Nonstick cooking spray
1 pint blackberries
2 tablespoons sugar
1 cup thawed frozen reduced-fat nondairy
   whipped topping
1 container (6 ounces) custard-style apricot or
   peach low-fat yogurt

1. Preheat oven to 400°F. Cut each sheet of phyllo crosswise into 4 pieces. Coat 1 piece lightly with cooking spray; place in large custard cup. Coat remaining 3 pieces lightly with cooking spray; place over first piece, alternating corners. Repeat with remaining phyllo dough to form 6 strudel cups.

2. Place custard cups on cookie sheet. Bake about 15 minutes or until pastry is golden. Let cool to room temperature.

3. Meanwhile, combine blackberries and sugar in small bowl; let stand 15 minutes.

4. Combine whipped topping and yogurt in medium bowl. Reserve ½ cup blackberries for garnish; gently stir remaining blackberries into whipped topping mixture. Spoon into cooled pastry cups. Top with reserved blackberries. Garnish with mint, if desired.

Makes 6 servings

NUTRIENTS PER SERVING:

Calories	126	Dietary Fiber	3 g
% calories from fat	22	Protein	3 g
Total Fat	4 g	Calcium	55 mg
Saturated Fat	<1 g	Iron	<1 mg
Cholesterol	3 mg	Vitamin A	25 RE
Sodium	22 mg	Vitamin C	10 mg
Carbohydrate	25 g		

Dietary Exchanges per Serving: 1½ Fruit, 1 Fat

Health Tip: Blackberries are a great source of fiber—two thirds of the fiber is insoluble, which helps keep your digestive tract running smoothly.

Mocha Crinkles

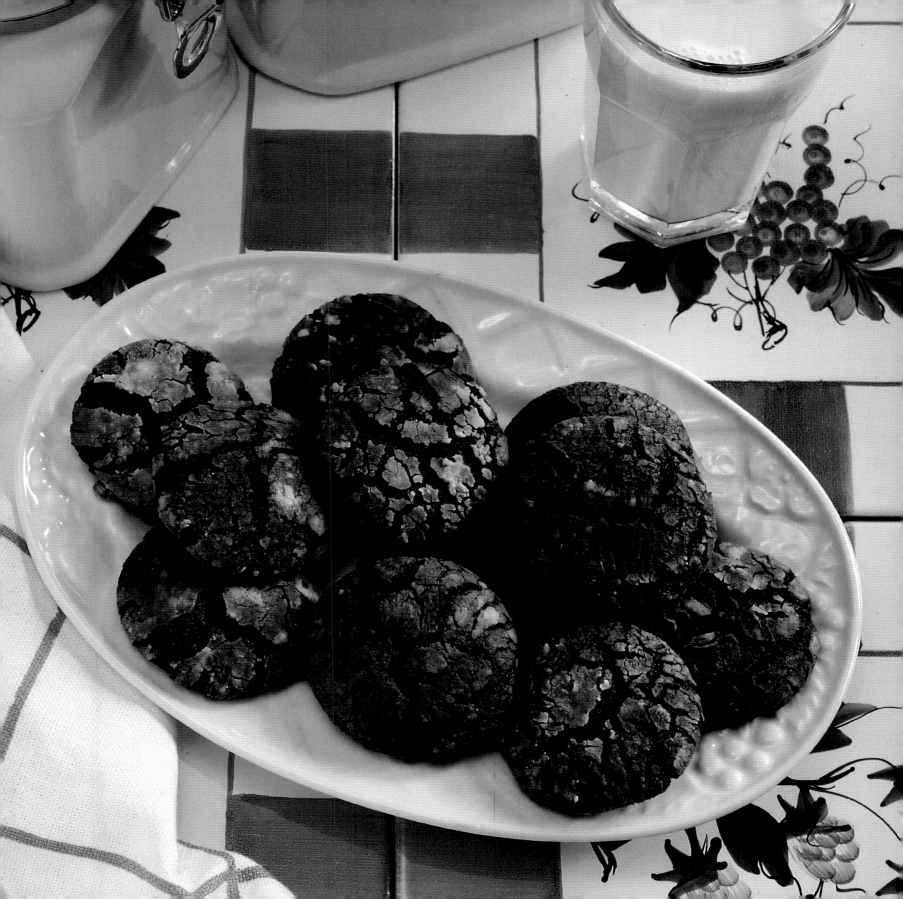

Raspberry-Applesauce Coffee Cake

1½ cups raspberries
¼ cup water
7 tablespoons sugar, divided
2 tablespoons cornstarch
½ teaspoon ground nutmeg, divided
1¾ cups all-purpose flour, divided
3 tablespoons margarine
1 tablespoon finely chopped walnuts
1½ teaspoons baking powder
½ teaspoon baking soda
⅛ teaspoon ground cloves
2 egg whites
1 cup unsweetened applesauce

1. Preheat oven to 350°F. Spray 8-inch square baking pan with nonstick cooking spray. Combine raspberries and water in small saucepan. Bring to a boil over high heat. Reduce heat to medium. Combine 2 tablespoons sugar, cornstarch and ¼ teaspoon nutmeg in small bowl. Stir into raspberry mixture. Cook and stir until mixture boils and thickens. Cook and stir 2 minutes more; set aside.

2. Combine ¾ cup flour and remaining 5 tablespoons sugar in medium bowl. Cut in margarine with pastry blender until mixture resembles coarse crumbs; set aside ½ cup crumb mixture for topping.

3. Add remaining 1 cup flour, walnuts, baking powder, baking soda, remaining ¼ teaspoon nutmeg and cloves to remaining crumb mixture. Add egg whites and applesauce; beat until well combined. Spread half of batter into prepared baking pan. Spread raspberry mixture over batter. Drop remaining batter into small mounds on top. Sprinkle with reserved topping.

4. Bake 40 to 45 minutes or until edges start to pull away from sides of pan. Serve warm or cool.

Makes 9 servings

NUTRIENTS PER SERVING:

Calories	196	Dietary Fiber	2 g
% calories from fat	21	Protein	4 g
Total Fat	5 g	Calcium	21 mg
Saturated Fat	1 g	Iron	1 mg
Cholesterol	0 mg	Vitamin A	50 RE
Sodium	158 mg	Vitamin C	6 mg
Carbohydrate	35 g		

Dietary Exchanges per Serving: 1 Starch/Bread, 1½ Fruit, 1 Fat

Raspberry-Applesauce Coffee Cake

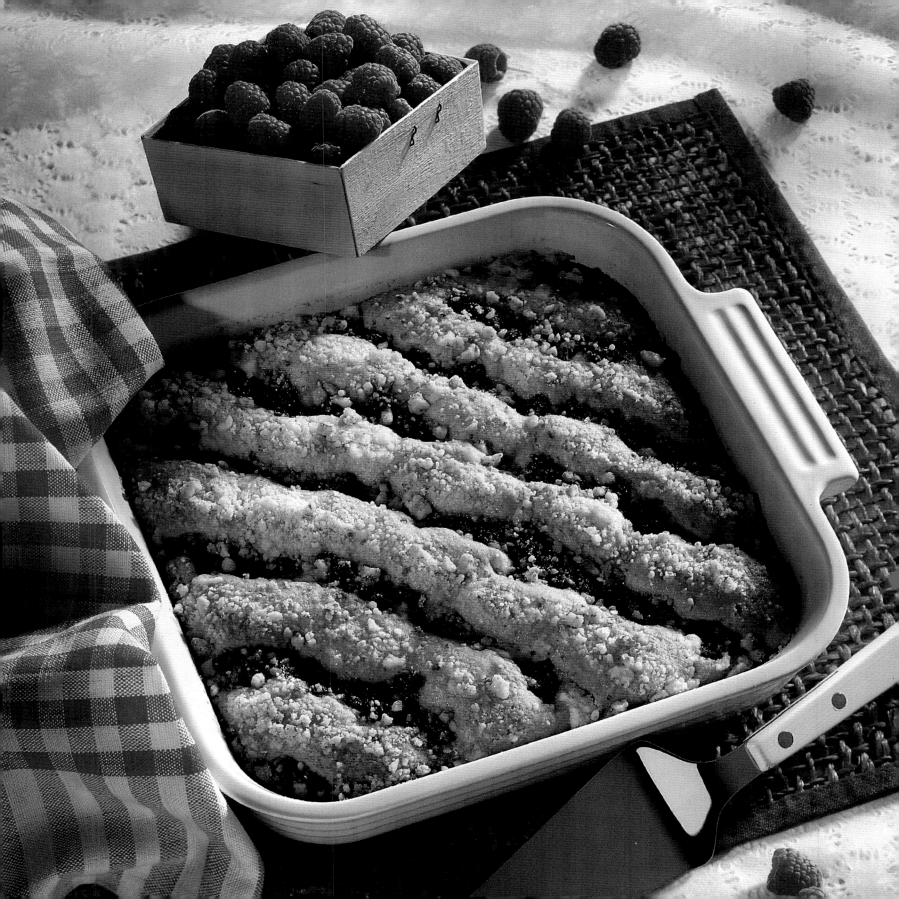

INDEX

METRIC CONVERSION CHART

VOLUME MEASUREMENTS (dry)

1/8 teaspoon = 0.5 mL
1/4 teaspoon = 1 mL
1/2 teaspoon = 2 mL
3/4 teaspoon = 4 mL
1 teaspoon = 5 mL
1 tablespoon = 15 mL
2 tablespoons = 30 mL
1/4 cup = 60 mL
1/3 cup = 75 mL
1/2 cup = 125 mL
2/3 cup = 150 mL
3/4 cup = 175 mL
1 cup = 250 mL
2 cups = 1 pint = 500 mL
3 cups = 750 mL
4 cups = 1 quart = 1 L

VOLUME MEASUREMENTS (fluid)

1 fluid ounce (2 tablespoons) = 30 mL
4 fluid ounces (1/2 cup) = 125 mL
8 fluid ounces (1 cup) = 250 mL
12 fluid ounces (1½ cups) = 375 mL
16 fluid ounces (2 cups) = 500 mL

WEIGHTS (mass)

1/2 ounce = 15 g
1 ounce = 30 g
3 ounces = 90 g
4 ounces = 120 g
8 ounces = 225 g
10 ounces = 285 g
12 ounces = 360 g
16 ounces = 1 pound = 450 g

DIMENSIONS

1/16 inch = 2 mm
1/8 inch = 3 mm
1/4 inch = 6 mm
1/2 inch = 1.5 cm
3/4 inch = 2 cm
1 inch = 2.5 cm

OVEN TEMPERATURES

250°F = 120°C
275°F = 140°C
300°F = 150°C
325°F = 160°C
350°F = 180°C
375°F = 190°C
400°F = 200°C
425°F = 220°C
450°F = 230°C

BAKING PAN SIZES

Utensil	Size in Inches/Quarts	Metric Volume	Size in Centimeters
Baking or Cake Pan (square or rectangular)	8×8×2	2 L	20×20×5
	9×9×2	2.5 L	22×22×5
	12×8×2	3 L	30×20×5
	13×9×2	3.5 L	33×23×5
Loaf Pan	8×4×3	1.5 L	20×10×7
	9×5×3	2 L	23×13×7
Round Layer Cake Pan	8×1½	1.2 L	20×4
	9×1½	1.5 L	23×4
Pie Plate	8×1¼	750 mL	20×3
	9×1¼	1 L	23×3
Baking Dish or Casserole	1 quart	1 L	—
	1½ quart	1.5 L	—
	2 quart	2 L	—